70 AND STRONG!

AGE IS NO BARRIER TO HEALTHY LIVING

WILL ANDERSON

CONTENTS

I dedicate this book to my dad.
-Will Anderson

FOREWORD

In the winter of 1965, my dad suffered a pretty serious heart attack. He was only 55. Back then, recovering from a heart attack meant lying in bed for two weeks or so, ostensibly to stabilize the heart muscle and allow it to heal.

While he was in hospital, my father contracted pneumonia, not uncommon for heart attack victims. He was in bad shape for several days until the antibiotics kicked in.

Once he was released, his doctor told him what he needed to do to enhance his recovery; new studies were beginning to show that exercising the heart muscle was generating amazing levels of healing and strengthening and patients were returning to full health faster. So, dad's first step was to get out of the house and start walking every day.

But it was winter and it was cold. North winds brought wind chills that were brutal and when Dad went out for those walks, he wouldn't get further than a hundred yards from our house before he began to feel angina pains in his chest. So, he'd simply turn around and come home.

Let me take a moment to describe my dad's lifestyle, which was similar to millions of men like him. He had an office job; he was a heavy smoker and in the mid-60s, everyone smoked. He had a fat-laden diet that consisted of lots of cheese, meat, and processed foods. His cholesterol was sky-high. He was clinically obese. His skin had a greyish hue. He never exercised unless you consider cutting the lawn or shovelling snow exercise, (it is but the wrong type!)

In short, my dad was a walking billboard for a heart attack waiting to happen.

His heart health continued to be unstable, largely because he never adopted a lifestyle that would correct it and, at the age of just 70, he died.

Today, of course, we know so much more about how to gain health and keep it. We know that smoking is a flat out killer. Everyone agrees that diet is an enormous contributor to an early death. Yet, heart disease and cancer (much of it due to smoking) are still the two main causes of death in North America.

Against this backdrop, demographics are playing an ever growing role; put simply, the population is aging. Fast. According to the Population Reference Bureau in the U.S., by 2040, one in five Americans will be 65 or older. That's less than 20 years from now! We cannot wait for the creaking, under-funded healthcare system to step in and look after us. We must manage that ourselves.

Stay Strong After 70! Is my attempt to put the power of healthy living back into our hands and show how we–not a strained Medicare or Medicaid system – are responsible for our own health.

INTRODUCTION

Welcome to the beginning of your health journey. If you've picked up this book, you have decided to make a commitment to better health. This is a profound step in the journey of your overall well-being. It is to be applauded. You have accepted the fact that age has crept up on you but you're not ready to give up on the vitality of your life. I have good news for you. Age is inevitable, but loss of vitality is not. You have a choice in the matter.

It wasn't too far back in our history that our life expectancies were considerably shorter but with modern science, the longevity of a human life has only grown. Though we'll go into that more in later chapters, it's important to understand that you don't have to fade away in your twilight years. Instead, you can seize this moment and begin to live a healthier, more fulfilling life. You can live a full life, filled with health and purpose, starting right now.

Too many think that it's too late to start their health journey when they are in their 60s or 70s. Fitness, they have decided, is a young man's game. This couldn't be further from the truth. At any age, you can begin making healthier choices that benefit you both physically and mentally. There is no reason to sit back and accept the toll time has taken on your body.

Taking control of your health, at any point in your life, opens the door to aging with grace and fulfillment. Yes, it's important to your overall health to begin eating healthier and exercising but you might also notice that your state of mind changes as well. You'll find more satisfaction in the day-to-day as you follow the steps in this book. You might even find that you have more energy, more enjoyment in the little things. This is all a natural part of the process.

In this book, we'll go over what it means to age—what it *really* means—and how you can bolster your health through healthy eating and low impact exercises. Eating healthy and exercising do not need to be taxing or expensive endeavors. This book was created to help you understand that it's about commitment, more than anything else. You will need to commit to a healthier lifestyle in order to reap the benefits.

Commitment is difficult. It necessitates that you make a choice every day to stick to your guns and continue with the decision that you have made. However, as you begin to implement the practices in this book, it will start to become habit. There is no truth in the adage that you can't teach an old dog new tricks. We are living in an ever changing world where old fogeys like us are learning new and exciting things every day. Because we're neither old nor fogeys. (Make this your mantra!)

This is your call to action. You have already taken the first step. You have picked up this book and begun reading. However, the most important step you can take is never the first one but the next one. So, it is important that you keep up that momentum, read on, and implement these practices into your every day. It might be a slow start but any movement is movement.

I wish you the best of luck in this endeavor. I have cultivated this book to make it easy for you. It is split up into helpful sections that cover everything from low impact exercises, what to avoid in the grocery store, and even what supplements may or may not be helpful. Furthermore, we'll take a look at what science currently says about aging and what the future of aging will look like for the typical person.

I commend you for making the time for your health. We are only granted one body in a lifetime and it is important that we understand exactly how to care for it so that we can spend as much time as we have with our loved ones. That's what this book is about, loving ourselves enough to take care of ourselves. I wish you the best of luck.

1

GROWING OLD DOES NOT MEAN GROWING WEAK

70 IS THE NEW 50

We've all heard it. Seventy is the new fifty. It has a nice ring to it, doesn't it? However, we rarely stop to think about what that actually *means*. It's not just a hip catchphrase. There's real science to back it up. We *have* made great strides in medical science that has shown us how to naturally prolong our lives. Seventy is no longer what it was. There is room for growth and development, even at this age.

So, why is seventy the new fifty? There are several reasons for this new sentiment, each of which give credence to the adage. First of all, due to advances in science, we are living longer than ever. Not too long ago, one might not expect to live past their 70s but with modern medicine and technology, this is no longer the case. We are living longer so the time to understand geriatric health is now.

Due to this relatively new longevity, those in their 60s and 70s are living active and healthy lives, assisted by modern medicine and current knowledge. There are several studies in this book that you might find enlightening and encouraging in your journey towards health. You might also find yourself with more energy and more drive to get out there and do more.

Many people in their twilight years are pushing off retirement, choosing to remain working in order to keep their minds and bodies active. This means that there is now room in the workforce for someone like you. Whether you choose to go this path or not is immaterial. What matters is that this is the new reality in which we live.

If you're not interested in remaining part of the workforce, there are plenty of other ways in which you can remain connected to your community. Volunteer opportunities are abundant in many areas and welcome those in their twilight years who are looking for ways to insert community and meaning into their every day life.

However you remain within the community, active and connected, you can add to the overall quality of life for those around you. Volunteering or working not only keeps your body and mind active, but better the community in which you live. You have so much to offer and the world is finally taking notice.

Because of this new reality, those in their seventies are being viewed differently. They are no longer viewed as those nearing the end of their life but as full members of the workforce, lively individuals, and most importantly, people of wisdom. This change of perspective means that life has taken on a whole new meaning for the aging population.

You have a lot to share as someone who has made it this far in life and you want to continue sharing that wealth of knowledge and wisdom. That is why it is so important that you take the time to focus on your health. You will, after all, be around for a while. Enjoy your stay by taking care of yourself in the best way possible.

This can be a major shift in how you view your life, which might feel uncomfortable at first. However, remember that you are in control of your own destiny and you call the shots. What you might need is a new outlook. Challenge what you have always believed and start living the active life of your dreams.

This can look like a lot of different things and we can address what your personal health journey will look like as we go through this book. However, it is important to address how your outlook can affect your progress and ultimate success. It's imperative that you have the right mindset as you tackle this new way of living.

CHANGING YOUR LIFE BY CHANGING YOUR OUTLOOK

When it comes to making this major change in your life, it all has to start in your mind and in your heart. You can no longer rely on old knowledge and outdated beliefs. It is time to change your outlook and better understand this new path you are on. You are capable of new growth. In fact, it is in your best interest to pursue it.

Later in this book, we will address all the reasons why staying active is vital to your quality of life. However, right now, you just need to know that it *is* important. There are many reasons to want to take the reins of your health journey. Whatever the reason, you can be confident that changing your outlook is a great first step.

So, why is it so important to change your outlook? After all, your current one has served you well thus far. For starters, it breaks you out of monotony. At any age, looking at things through a new lens can break the cycle of sameness. We want to see a concept from new angles, to fully understand the big picture.

It's okay if you look around and realize that somewhere along the line, you fell off the path that you had walked as a younger person. Life kept rolling and somewhere along the line, you looked back and realized that you put your health on a shelf to worry about later. It happens to the best of us.

However, you need to understand that your life is not over. You still have time to make changes in your life that will not only benefit yourself but those around you. You are taking the reins of your life and making decisions that will better yourself. That's a great step. Let's take a look at some of the benefits of challenging your current outlook. Aside from becoming a healthier you, these benefits include:

1. Bolstering your self-esteem
2. Enhancing your quality of life
3. Cultivating and strengthening relationships
4. Achieving a sense of accomplishment
5. Living your life with purpose

All of these reasons should be something that you keep in mind as you continue through your health journey. It is a mind-body experience, benefitting all parts of your life. You are on the path to inner healing through positive change. That is a commendable endeavor.

Now that I've regaled you with the positive aspects of changing your outlook on life and making health a priority, it's important to make a game plan. After all, habits take time to build and changing out the lens by which you see the world can seem like a daunting task. In order to tackle this, you want to have an idea of where you're headed so let's start with a simple five-step strategy.

Let's start by envisioning the changes you want to make in your life. Do you want to increase your stamina so you can spend more time chasing after the grandkids? Do you want to increase your strength so you are no longer wrestling with pickle jars? Do you want to begin a workout class to find community with others? These are all great aspirations. Having them clear in your mind is great but journaling them out and really seeing them for what they are is important as well. Take five minutes to write about your health aspirations.

Next, you want to do some soul searching to understand why

these things are important to you. Perhaps you haven't been able to keep up with the grandkids in a while. Maybe you are lonely and wish to seek out others through fitness classes. Whatever the reason, the whole journey takes on new meaning and purpose once you fully understand it.

Okay, you have the meaning behind your journey all figured out. That's a great place to start. Now, you want to do some planning for next steps. Make an action-plan on how you are going to accomplish your goals. For now, maybe it just looks like taking a brisk walk around the neighborhood every morning or signing up for a water aerobics class. You don't have to have it all figured out, but start making some plans!

You might start to notice that your excitement and momentum pick up speed once you start making plans. You really want to revisit your earlier journaling during this phase, as it will help you maintain your focus and drive. Look at your goals and look at what you need to do to get there. Soon enough, you'll see a clear path. This book is here to help you find that path.

Finally, make sure you keep up this visualization. Whenever you don't want to go on that morning walk, visualize yourself chasing after the grandkids. Whenever you don't feel like going to the gym, imagine yourself as part of a community, dedicated to a common goal. Imagining yourself at your personal "finish line" will allow you to really understand what you're striving for. It will make all the hard work seem oh-so-worth it.

CHALLENGING YOUR INNER CRITIC

Now, all of this is well and fine, you might be thinking. But doubt is creeping into your mind and already telling you that you are not capable of this type of change. This is your inner critic and it has no place in this journey. Aside from safety concerns, which we will go over in full detail, you should not be nay-saying this fitness journey.

You *do* have what it takes. However, I understand the feelings of doubt. I had them myself when I began writing this book. Whenever we strike out and start a new project, that little voice of self-doubt is crystal clear in our minds. The trick is, you don't have to listen to it. I will walk you through some great ways to silence that inner critic so that you are coming at this with all of your ability.

First, we need to take a look at how ageism plays into our own views on aging. We might realize that what we 'believe' about ourselves has really been an idea implanted in our mind through societal conditioning. In a recent survey done by the World Health Organization (WHO), it was discovered that the lowest rates of respect for elders were pooled in countries with higher incomes (Breeding, 2018). You read that right. The more well off a country is, the less they respect their elders.

This may or may not come as a surprise to you. However, you need to understand how this can play into how you view your own process of aging. If the society around you has a negative outlook on aging, it's likely that you have internalized that and have viewed aging with a measure of dread. Simply put, you're letting others dictate how you feel about your own aging process.

However, in many cultures around the world, old age is seen as a beautiful gift. Elders are viewed as wise and strong. They are looked after by the community and valued for their experience. Keep this in mind as you view your own aging process. You still have much to offer this world. You have a unique experience that is needed in this world.

Secondly, we need to do away with the concept that growing old means that our health must deteriorate. Though there might be genetic factors to contend with when it comes to overall health, you can still live a healthy and fulfilled life in your 70s, aging with the utmost of grace. There are those who have taken to this idea and created what is known as the positive aging movement.

Positive aging, simply put, is to view aging as a normal and natural part of life, embracing it for what it is. It is welcoming aging instead of shunning the beginning signs of it. It is a movement of radical acceptance. It is also the commitment that you will continue to whatever needs to be done in order to continue enjoying the things you have always enjoyed. That means, yes, taking control of your health so that you are still able to take joy in your hobbies as you age. It all ties in together.

Finally, you really just need to understand your limitations and your goals and have a can-do spirit. It sounds trite, but it's the beginning of most endeavors—believing you have what it takes. You have made it this far in your life so I have no doubt that you have the tenacity and determination necessary to make this work. Tell that little annoying critic in your brain that he or she doesn't get to determine your grit or your worth. You are in control of your own health journey.

That being said, you want to curb your expectations. You might be able to achieve certain goals but try not to shoot for the moon. They aren't recruiting 70-year-old NBA players so maybe strike that from your list. Do the exercises that feel right for your goals and your passions and you should be on the right track.

THE BOTTOM LINE

Knowing is half the battle, or so says G.I. Joe. However, this adage is not without its merit. Starting your journey with the right knowledge and mindset is a stepping stone to success. By challenging your own misconceptions about age, you are working toward a more fulfilled life. Don't let your negative inner voice talk you out of this, and don't let society dictate what you are capable of.

You get to decide how this journey begins. So take some time to really get to know yourself and your reasons for wanting to pursue fitness. It is important to have that driving force behind you as you work towards better physical health. Of course, it is also important to understand what current studies are saying about the connection between remaining active and the aging practice.

While the world waits with bated breath to see how the systemic issues of the struggling health care system will handle the growing needs of the population, we can take personal responsibility for our own health. Staying fit and healthy into our twilight years will assuage a bit of that burden. Furthermore, it will save us money and struggle in the long term. So consider how you are going to take care of yourself as you age. It can make all the difference. The next chapter will venture into that territory, giving you a better picture of what to expect from the future of healthcare and how it will affect you.

2

THE HEALTHCARE SYSTEM AND AGING

As we discuss your own personal health journey, it's also important to see the bigger picture. The current healthcare system has not adjusted well to a rapidly aging population living longer and this has caused difficulties throughout the years. While we are taking personal responsibility for our own health, we must also understand the bigger implications.

THE IMPLICATIONS OF A HEALTHIER ELDERLY POPULATION

The healthcare system in the US has been a topic of hot debate for some time. The expense of healthcare is a heavy burden that has strained budgets at the federal, state, county, and individual levels for decades. When considering the topic of this book, we must also consider what it would mean for healthcare as a whole.

With the population living longer, there is a heavier burden on the healthcare system to care for aging adults. However, if we can find a way to improve the health of the older population through staying active and eating right, we can reduce a great deal of pressure on the mainstream system.

The world of healthcare will be forever changed as more people live longer. According to a report presented by the World Health Organization (WHO), "the number of people aged 65 or older is projected to grow from an estimated 524 million in 2010 to nearly 1.5 billion in 2050" (Garza 2016). On the one hand, this growth of the elderly population is good news, because we are living longer. On the other hand, it creates its own new and unique challenges for healthcare:

- A need for more resources like long-term critical care homes and geriatric doctors across all health care settings
- An ever-increasing need to battle against obesity
- A growing shortage of healthcare workers
- The diversity of health care providers is lagging behind the growing diversity of patients
- Changes in family structures may lead to fewer family caregivers

Let's take a look at each of these issues in more detail. It can help us better understand the current state of US healthcare and what it might mean for you in the future.

1. An increased need for resources across all healthcare settings is probably one of the more concerning factors to consider. We are at a crossroads, where it has become imperative that more resources be allocated to the US healthcare system. This is not something that we, as individuals, can affect directly but we *can* make our legislators stand up and listen to us. So, let your voice be

heard and pay close attention to who is taking up the call to get this done.

2. Obesity, however, is one area that you have direct control over, if only for yourself. Though you can't stop the rise of the problem, you can control your own eating habits. The section of this book that covers healthy eating should act as a great blueprint for you to sidestep this particular issue. Pay close attention to the scale and eliminate empty calories from your diet to keep yourself in the clear.

3. There *is* a growing shortage of healthcare workers, which can spell disaster not just for geriatric care but for health care in general. This can greatly impact the nation's ability to see to the health of the population. With people living longer, there is a greater strain at a time when we are seeing fewer individuals enter the medical field. This is a problem that should be addressed through legislation and special initiatives.

4. Here is where it gets sticky. The diversity of health care workers is currently lagging behind the diversity of the population. This means that many patients are not being adequately represented by those who are caring for them. The best thing you can do for yourself here is to stick with your new healthy lifestyle and adequately address issues with your primary care provider.

5. Changes in the typical family structure constitute one of the factors influenced by current culture. No longer are adults taking care of their aging family members. They don't have the time or the resources to do so. Every household has to be a two- income household and there is no one left at home to care for the aging. This means that there is more need for good, assisted living environments.

In order for the health care system to truly tackle the aging population, ways must be found to address these problems. However, as individuals, we can be part of the solution, rather than part of the problem. Through careful living—staying active and eating right—we can reduce the need for care by reducing preventable illnesses. Put simply, through mindful living, we can lessen the strain on the healthcare system.

Proper nutrition and exercise can decrease your health care needs, taking some of the weight off of the system. Though it will not completely solve the problem, it will free up the resources necessary to care for the aging population. We are not responsible for solving systemic issues in the healthcare system, but we can take accountability for our own health.

WHY YOU SHOULD BE VISITING A DOCTOR

You *should* be seeing your primary care provider. They can keep you apprised of your current health and any possible points of concern. While eating healthy and staying active are important factors in keeping your body in tip top shape, your doctor can also advise you on any concerns you might have.

Even though the healthcare system is overburdened, that does not mean you should stop seeing your doctor. Instead, be mindful when you visit. Write down any questions you may have in advance. Sometimes, in the moment, we can forget what we wanted to ask.

Furthermore, understand what your needs are. Navigating health insurance and copays can be difficult but if you find that you are not having your needs met by a certain provider, then it might be time to move on to someone who is listening to your concerns. These doctors are the ones who will help you maintain and develop good health strategies.

Having a good primary care provider can ensure that you are on the right track with your health journey. Under their guidance you will find that you can achieve more than if you were to go it alone. They can help you avoid health pitfalls and advise you on genetic disorders that you might want to look out for. Having this advocate in your corner is something that can only benefit your health goals.

Furthermore, you might want to run some of the practices in this book by them. They might have some ideas of their own on what would be the best exercises and dietary needs for your current health. This book can only go so far and health is not one-size-fits-all. Therefore, having a great primary care provider can go a long way in helping you achieve your health goals. Furthermore, regular check-ups can keep you out of the assisted living facilities that are currently under fire for reasons that we will go into in the next section of this chapter.

LONG-TERM CARE FACILITIES

Long-term care facilities are an eventuality for many aging adults. Due to the changing family dynamics discussed earlier in this chapter, more and more families are opting to place their elderly in assisted living and long-term care facilities. After all, not many households have the ability to care for someone anymore, with long hours and shrinking wages.

Long-term care facilities have notoriously high turnover rates in staff, and with an ever-growing crisis regarding the number of health care professionals in the field, this has led to many issues in these facilities. For starters, the COVID pandemic hit nursing homes and assisted living facilities hard. A large proportion of the fatal cases took place within the walls of such facilities.

Furthermore, infection has begun to be a real issue in long-term facilities. Many of the deaths that occur in long-term care facilities can be traced back to some type of infection. Because of the growing shortage of health care workers, many staff members are pulling longer shifts and the consequences of exhaustion can be dire for those under their care.

My intention is not to scare you but to apprise you of the issues that face a lot of these facilities. For this reason, you want to maintain your independence as long as you can, making your health a priority. However, should you find yourself in one of these facilities sooner rather than later, keep yourself informed of the issues facing your particular residence. You will want to be your own best advocate for your health.

The best way to mitigate the need for long term care is to stay active and stay on top of your health. Those who live an active lifestyle are less likely to find themselves in need of assisted living facilities such as these. To maintain your mobility and independence, you will want to stay active, eat right, practice proper sleep hygiene, and take care of your mental health, too. These are all important factors when addressing your overall health and the length of time that you can be independent.

THE BOTTOM LINE

While it might not be fun to consider the current and future landscape of US health care, it is necessary to understand it. You want to know what to expect and the unique concerns facing aging individuals in this equation. While there are many things that can only be addressed by legislation and systemic changes, you can still keep yourself healthy and knowledgeable.

It bears repeating that it is still important that you visit your primary care provider on a regular basis so that you can remain apprised of any health concerns that you might be facing. Furthermore, it is helpful in your current health journey to have an advocate in your corner—someone who can direct you in the best way to take control of your health.

Assisted living facilities are seeing a decline in health care workers joining their ranks which, in turn, has created a shortage of workers and an increase in infections facing residents.

Of course, the best outcome would be avoiding these facilities altogether. The best way to mitigate the possibility is to keep yourself healthy, through active living and healthy eating. I know I have harped on this point a lot but my intention is to really drive the point home.

The healthcare system is not the only thing you should keep your eye on. There are also promising studies in the future of aging that can give you hope for the journey ahead and can act as a road map as you navigate through your unique health challenges. The next chapter highlights some of these studies and what they mean for your health journey.

3

<hr>

WHAT CURRENT STUDIES SAY ABOUT AGING

When starting a health journey of this sort, it is important to understand what the experts have to say. This chapter will be a brief overview of some of the latest studies in aging and how they will impact your game plan. Pay close attention to what these experts have to say, as their research is the foundation for much of the helpful practices in this book.

STAYING ACTIVE IS PROLONGING YOUR LIFE

We all know that staying active is more than just looking good in a set of joggers. Working out has tremendous benefits for the body and mind, ranging from lowered inflammation to bolstered levels of serotonin. However, what you might not realize is that these benefits are helping you fight back against Father Time.

Everyone wants extra time. Whether it's to pursue our passions or to spend more time with our loved ones, we all seem to want just a little bit more of the grains of sand in life's hourglass. Studies have been done on how remaining active impacts the longevity of a human life, and the news is good!

Let's take a look at a study that we all might have some passing familiarity with—the Dallas Bed Rest and Training Study. In this study, five healthy young men were selected for an assignment that sounded like a dream. They merely had to spend three of their summer weeks in bed, remaining sedentary for the entire length of their time there. However, the young men did not bank on the outcome of the study which was devastating in its revelations.

All of the young men who participated in the study were tested before and after exercise once their three weeks were up. The results shocked even the researchers in its ramifications—a faster resting heart rate, a rise in body fat, higher systolic blood pressure, a significant drop in the heart's maximum pumping capacity, and a measurable fall in muscle strength.

In just three weeks of remaining sedentary, these 20-somethings had developed many physiological traits of men twice their age. The results of this were clear but the scientists took it one step further. Following the period of bed rest and the subsequent testing, the researchers entered the young men in an 8-week exercise program. The results were fantastic. Not only were the results of the initial study reversed, but many of the men came out of it with better results than they'd had *prior* to joining the study.

What we can take from this is that remaining stagnant in our health journey is taking a real toll on our bodies. These men showed signs of deterioration after a mere three weeks of remaining sedentary. Submitting yourself to age and staying in place can do serious damage to your health. Alternatively, maintaining a regular exercise routine can reverse these effects.

You might be asking, however, does this really lengthen your life span? While it's true that there are genetic factors that can leave you more predisposed to certain health risks, these benefits can combat many of the major health problems that end a life. Heart disease and stroke are far less likely to occur when you are maintaining good cardiovascular health through active exercise.

Furthermore, there was a correlation between cardiovascular health and longevity found in a study conducted by *JAMA (Journal of the American Medical Association)*. In simplest terms, they were looking to explore the association between long-term mortality and levels of cardiovascular fitness. What they discovered was both fascinating and optimistic.

Cardiovascular fitness is a measure of how well your heart and lungs output blood and oxygen to the rest of your body. This measure can be greatly improved through regular exercise and eating right. In order to study the correlation between this measure and how long a person lives, the researchers pooled data from over 122,000 patients at a medical center who underwent exercise testing on a treadmill, an objective test of cardiovascular fitness.

According to the findings of this study, longer living was associated with higher levels of cardiovascular fitness. This means that keeping that blood pumping with good exercise and clean eating can greatly impact the number of years that you spend with your loved ones. With something so simple having such a great impact, it is important to take notice.

Furthermore, the proof is in our very DNA. Results of a Brigham Young University research initiative were very telling about the correlation between regular exercise and longer lifetimes. Researchers at Brigham Young studied the DNA of 6,000 adults and what they found was remarkable.

First, a lesson in DNA. There are end caps to DNA called telomeres that shorten with age. However, what these BYU researchers discovered was that active adults in their pool had longer telomeres than those who lived a sedentary lifestyle. This equates to about a 9 year difference in cell age in those who were active versus those who were not.

Another study found that the lungs and hearts of 70 year old males who were active were in far greater shape than those who were more sedentary. Wherever you look, the proof is evident. Staying active can greatly impact the length of your life. With all this evidence, it should be an encouragement to get up and start exercising regularly.

The evidence is damning for those who live a sedentary lifestyle. There is an urgent need to take control of your health by implementing healthy exercise into your routine. With the ample evidence mounting as more and more studies come out, you can no longer deny that living a sedentary lifestyle is impractical when wanting to live a longer life. Not just impractical, but dangerous.

Exercising daily—even low impact exercises—can make a world of difference to your cardiovascular fitness. Thus, you could be looking at a longer and healthier life. Making this change can be hard but knowing this, it's impossible not to put importance on fitness at this time in your life. It's now, more than ever, that your health is a priority and taking the reins could mean all the difference.

Now, you might be saying, exercise is a young man's game. You might already be feeling the effects of an aging body. However, there are low impact exercises you can do from the comfort of your own neighborhood, or even your own living room, that can make all the difference in your overall health. You just need some guidance on what that might look like.

As mentioned before, you can try taking up a brisk walk every day. It's a great way to get moving and get that blood pumping. You don't need to run a marathon for the exercise to be effective. Furthermore, you can try low impact exercises like swimming, or even lifting small weights for strength training. We will go into proper exercises in chapter 4, but for now, know that they exist and you can change—and lengthen—your life by staying active.

COGNITIVE BENEFITS OF MAKING HEALTH A PRIORITY

Aside from the remarkable physical benefits of exercise and eating, one must also consider the cognitive benefits. After all, it is often believed that age dulls the mind. However, recent science calls into question whether this need be the case. In fact, it seems that those who decide to live active lives are less likely to see a decline of their mental status as they age.

Cognitive functioning typically refers to a number of different mental abilities, including but not contained to, thinking, language, learning, and concentration. Though these might all seem like the same function, they all actually originate from different parts of the brain, making them smaller parts of a larger whole. Cognitive functioning has been known to degrade as one ages. However, there are measures you can take to ensure that your mental faculties remain the best that they can be.

While several theoretical and empirical studies have reported that cognitive functioning declines with age, there is hope. Due to the fact that humans are living longer than ever before, the study of these cognitive declines has been a point of interest for medical studies. What they have found is optimistic in nature. There are several studies that have looked at the decline of mental faculties in aging and their results were promising.

For instance, let's look at a particular study conducted in Chicago recently. This study was simple in its structure. It measured how often a subject stood or sat and then took a look at that person's brain after they had passed away. In doing this, they hoped to measure how remaining active could influence the brain's activity and structure. Their findings were both crucial and eye-opening.

What they found, while taking a look at the brains of the deceased, was that certain immune cells worked entirely differently in those elderly who had been more active compared to their sedentary peers. Physical activity not only positively affected their cognitive functioning, but changed how diseases like Alzheimer's affected them—whether or not they experienced memory loss. This study just adds to growing evidence that working out our bodies is paying off for our minds as well.

This is not the only study that points to cognitive benefits of regular physical activity. It has been shown that older, more sedentary people in their 70s and up can add volume to their hippocampus by walking for just an hour a day. This is important, as the hippocampus is the brain's memory center. No more forgetting where your keys are located. Just keep up your regularly scheduled walk.

This is not to say that genetics does not play a part, as we have gone over previously. There is still a possibility of active adults developing genetic memory disorders such as Alzheimer's. However, it has been noted that the onset typically happens years later in active people and the symptoms are much less pronounced in the patients. So though you might not be able to outrun genetics, you can slow down the progression of certain disorders that target your mental faculties and take the reins, so to speak. You might not get to decide your genetics, but you have a say in how the disorder plays out in the long term.

There's even more evidence that backs up this correlation, as middle-aged and elderly people are more likely to do well on tests of memory and thinking skills. This is good news for those choosing to embark on a fitness journey of their own. Though the reasoning behind this correlation is still somewhat of a medical mystery, the proof is in the pudding. Staying active has remarkable effects on the very shape and functioning of your brain. So, keep at it!

This goes back to choosing to start this health journey to continue doing the things you love. If you enjoy things that require mental activity, then this is your reason to stay active. Exercise will be your best friend as you strive to keep that mind sharp. So, you can continue reading your mystery novels and solving them before you turn that last page. Alternately, you can continue crushing your grandkids in Words With Friends. Whatever your hobby may be, if it requires cognitive functioning, you will only see this improve as you become more active.

FOOD RESTRICTIONS (NOT CALORIE RESTRICTIONS)

There are way too many diet books out there. I will not add to the noise. You don't need to worry about counting calories and eating based on the most recent fad diet. This is not, after all, about shedding pounds. It's about knowing how to eat healthy in order to live your most fulfilled life. There are things you need to take into consideration that you might not have thought much about in your youth. I will walk you through the basic science of what that might look like for you.

This means that you will have a better understanding of how things like appetite and calorie intake affect your body and mind. You want to pay attention to the foods you're eating because they are inextricably linked to your current wellbeing. There are certain things to consider that you might not realize as you grow older.

For instance, something that might surprise you is that the feeling of thirst declines as you age. Keeping this in mind, you will want to watch your fluid intake. Make sure that you are getting enough hydration, especially as you become more physically active. Hydration is an important part of the body's functioning so drink plenty of water. Set a daily reminder for yourself if necessary.

Secondly, you will want to eat a variety of foods. It can be easy to get stuck in our ways and continue eating the same thing that is comforting to us. However, variety is key when you are attempting to eat healthy. Not only does it break you out of the routine of unhealthy eating, but a balanced diet is a must as you age. We will go into more detail in chapter 5, but a healthy meal should consist of lean protein, fruits and veggies, dairy, and whole grains. There are ways to work all of these into your daily meal plan without breaking the bank. You just have to be savvy.

Due to the fact that you are now attempting to eat a variety of healthy foods, it might help to plan out meals. What can be daunting at first will become easier as you get into the swing of things. It can also take a lot of the guesswork out of your commitment to health. Consider creating a meal plan for the week and posting it on your refrigerator to refer back to. This can keep you on the right track.

Here's a tip that might be challenging: put away the table salt. As you age, your flavor receptors become more dulled and this can lead you to overdoing it on the salt. Watch your sodium intake as you age. Too much of a good thing is, in fact, a bad thing. Too much sodium in the diet can negatively impact your heart health.

Instead of reaching for the salt, consider shaking things up a little with some herbs and spices. They will add flavor to your meals without the added sodium. Fresh is best but you can also find these flavorful herbs stocked at your local grocery store. Some healthy alternatives to salt include cayenne pepper, sage, basil, and turmeric. (We will touch on turmeric in more detail in chapter 5, but needless to say, this one should definitely be in your pantry if it isn't already. Not only can these add much needed flavor to your dishes, but they will make you less likely to rely on salt for seasoning.

Alright, I know I just hit you where it hurts with the salt but I'm about to sucker punch you with another tough pill to swallow. You will want to start limiting your sugar intake. I know this one can be one of the hardest to follow. It is remarkable how much of our everyday foods are packed with sugar. However, you don't need to necessarily cut out sugar entirely. Just stray away from foods that are notorious for their high sugar count. Instead of reaching for a Snack Pack, consider substituting with natural treats like fruit, yams, or sweet peppers.

The cold hard truth is that obesity and diabetes have been a problem plaguing the geriatric community for some time. You can mitigate your risk of both issues by simply watching your sugar intake or, more drastically, deciding to do without altogether. Sugar wreaks havoc on the cells of the body and if you want to lengthen the lifetime of a cell, you want to walk away from the M&Ms and start reaching for more healthy, whole foods that satiate that sweet tooth like fresh fruits.

Finally, let's talk fats. There has been a lot of traction for no-fat diets over the years but you need not restrict yourself that much. Instead of cutting out fat altogether, try to stick to healthy fats. They are necessary to a balanced diet and can benefit you in the long run. Foods that are rich in healthy fats include olive oil, avocados, nuts, and fish that are high in omega-3 fatty acids. Sticking to these fats will keep you satisfied while keeping your heart health on the upswing.

THE BOTTOM LINE

The fact is, we can no longer plead ignorance about the correlation between exercising/healthy eating and a longer, healthier life. There is a mountain of evidence from recent studies that shows the effects of these factors on overall health. Not only will you benefit physically from making these changes in your lifestyle. You will also begin to see cognitive benefits.

A sedentary lifestyle with unhealthy eating habits is not serving you. If you want the extra time to spend with your loved ones, it is time to make the sacrifices necessary. This means opening the door to new experiences. However, with the right dedication, you will see some remarkable results in your life. The health benefits are worth the sacrifices.

Of course, as you start this journey, it's important to come to terms with the process of aging. We touched on it earlier in this book but understanding the aging process and what it looks like in other cultures can give you a broader understanding of your experience. We'll dive into that in the next chapter.

4

OLD AGE DOES NOT EQUAL WEAKNESS

As you age, you might start feeling like you have been pushed aside. This can make you feel weak and out of control. However, this need not be the case. You are a valuable part of the human race who deserves to live a healthy, fulfilling life. It's imperative that you understand this. Therefore, we will examine what this looks like in action.

WHY ELDERS MATTER

As mentioned earlier in this book, countries with higher income tend to treat their elderly with less respect. It's a documented phenomenon but it does not have to color your view of the world or, more importantly, yourself. Elders are important in our society, whether that is recognized or not.

There is one culture in particular we can learn from. The Indigenous people of North America are renowned for the respect they show their elders who are often the last tether to their cultural past. They continue the spoken and written history of their respective peoples. By taking a look at this culture, we can learn a thing or two about how to view ourselves in this aging process.

Think of it like this: you are like the root of the tree that is humankind. You are the basis of the traditions and values that have been passed down through generations. With your experiences, you have helped others understand the importance of things like family, working hard, and the value of a dollar.

Elders are ideal candidates for mentors Because of your accumulated experience and knowledge, you can look at a situation with objectivity and give constructive feedback to your children. And perhaps, their children. You are often the anchor of the family, keeping those around you connected, through your wisdom and through your persistence.

I know that I have often looked to my elders for guidance in times of trouble. After all, those older than me have lived more life than me. They understand what it is to walk through the hard times. That is something you can offer those around you. You have walked through the hard times and come out the other side. Your resilience in the face of adversity is something not only commendable but worth being shared.

Furthermore, you carry with you the traditions of your culture, whatever they may be. Without your knowledge of these customs, many of them would have died out. So take comfort in the fact that you are the embodiment of your culture, there to inspire younger generations. You might not think that it is a lot to offer but it is sad to see cultures forgotten. Carrying on the legacy can keep those cultures alive in the hearts and minds of generations to come.

Of course, there is also the fact that you have lived a lot of life. This is not just about wisdom but about learning how to appreciate yourself. You have walked this earth a long time and found what works to find fulfillment and what does not. You can pass this knowledge on, denouncing all the fretting and worrying that is happening around you. You have learned, through your years of experience, how to really suck the marrow out of life.

All of these are good reasons to respect yourself that you might be denied in your culture. However, the most important part of accepting your importance is understanding that you have inherent value as a human being. You don't have to be put on a shelf now, just because you have grown old. You deserve your place in this world. Your unique outlook and wisdom are just a few things you can offer as the incredible individual that you are, along with passion and love. And all of this is within you.

STRENGTH BEYOND THE PHYSICAL

As mentioned above, your strength is not all about physical capability. You might feel weak and feeble as you are entering your elder years. Though you are working on combating this, you might want to consider all the ways in which you are strong that have nothing to do with physical activity. For starters, you have made it this far in life. You have learned and grown as a human being, and that is a feat in and of itself.

Furthermore, lean into that wisdom that I mentioned in the section above. Your accumulated knowledge of the world puts you in a unique position to offer some tough pills to swallow. You have seen the world turn more times than the average person and you have a unique outlook to offer.

That's not to say that wisdom is all you have to offer. You also have joy. But first, you will need to cultivate that joy in yourself. I maintain that physical wellness is extremely important but it is important to consider the whole picture, the whole person. That means taking care of your mental health as well.

Sometimes, the term "mental health" can seem a bit buzzy. It is talked about often in today's society and it starts to lose its meaning as it is repeated over and over. However, mental health is vitally important to your overall well-being. We will go into more detail in a later chapter but for now, I will leave you with this, you only get one life and you want to spend that life happy and fulfilled.

This does not necessarily mean going to one of those hippie dippy yoga retreats and going vegan. However, there are practical mental health routines that you can implement that will greatly impact your everyday mental wellness. You just have to have the fortitude to make that commitment.

POWERING THROUGH

You might be reading this and begin to feel overwhelmed. This is natural when making a big change, good or otherwise. But I promise you, this journey will only benefit you in the long term. Still, you might be struggling to find momentum as you walk through these steps. That's where drawing on your own innate power is necessary.

You have a can-do spirit. It is evident just by the fact that you picked up this book. You *want* to make a change. Still, you might need some extra encouragement along the way. We've discussed telling our inner critic to shut up but what happens when it is the endless new routines that leave us feeling exhausted?

I won't lie to you. There will undoubtedly be obstacles as you walk down this path. You just need to know how to navigate around them. For starters, go back to the journaling you did at the beginning of this book. Envision your goals as you work through these obstacles. Having your endgame in mind can combat some of that dread of making these drastic changes. When you have a better understanding of why you are making these changes, you will have a better chance of achieving your goals.

So, take a moment to return to your reasoning for making these changes. Whatever the purpose behind your new health journey, you are looking for something at the finish line. Whatever that is, hold onto it. It will be the fire beneath your feet that keeps you running (figuratively speaking). You have the fire within you to make this work, you just need to keep reminding yourself of the stakes and the outcomes. This will keep you on the straight and narrow as you continue making the right health decisions for yourself.

You have what it takes to make these changes. You have made it this far in life, which is already an accomplishment. You have faced trials before and the obstacles you might face—like self-doubt, frustration, or setbacks—are not insurmountable. You just have to remember that you are a force to be reckoned with and push through the discomfort of these changes.

It's important to understand that these changes are necessary in maintaining your overall health and that powering through any challenges is just part of the process. You will start to become more confident in yourself as you progress through this journey but for now, just know that you have what it takes. You *can* do this. Moreover, you *should* be doing this. For yourself and for those you love.

MAKING THE COMMITMENT

It is my hope that, at this juncture, you fully understood the importance of this health journey. There are a great many benefits to taking control of your health and making it a priority. However, it can still be difficult to make a commitment to something so different from what you are used to. It can be hard to turn a desire into a habit.

We are creatures of habit, and if you have been somewhat sedentary, it can be hard to break out of that cycle and gain momentum. Furthermore, eating healthy can be a truly difficult task when you have fallen into a habit of eating as you please. Still, there are practices you can implement that will help you stick it out and create healthier habits for yourself.

We discussed understanding *why* you are making this commitment and reminding yourself of that whenever you need to. That part has undoubtedly been cemented in your mind. Great, that's the first step toward your health goals. However, you likely need practical help with how to keep to those goals.

The first thing you need to do is remove choice from the equation. If you have food in the house that you know you have a tendency to overindulge in, especially sugary treats, toss them out. Keep to a predetermined grocery list. Make a workout date with a friend or sign up for a prepaid class. Make sure that you have set things up in such a way that you are fully committed to showing up and staying healthy.

Furthermore, make sure your whole heart is in it. This goes back to keeping your goal in mind. With the right motivation, you can overcome your obstacles. You want to be fully in this. Show up for yourself, every day, with everything you have. Don't hold back any of that determination and grit that you have within yourself. Understand the importance of this journey and keep your mind open to changes.

In that same vein, question why you might not be coming at this with everything you have. What is holding you back? Perhaps journaling about some of the challenges can help you get a handle on the emotions you are feeling. Understand your obstacles better so you have a better chance at overcoming them.

Finally, consider taking small steps at first. I get it. You want to do everything all at once. This is all new information and you want to tackle everything in full go. However, that's a good way to burn yourself out. Start with small things you can change right now. Perhaps start by eliminating those sugary treats and work your way up from there. As far as exercise, perhaps just start with a daily walk to get that blood pumping. Whatever first step you take, fully commit to it and then build up from there. You will be surprised how easy it becomes to slowly add components of healthy living when you start small. Remember the old adage, "By the inch, it's a cinch. But by the yard, it is hard."

Whenever starting something new, you want to dip your toe in the water first, so to speak. You want to ensure that you are moving at a comfortable pace. Though you want to occasionally push yourself, doing too much at once can be overwhelming and cause you to burn out quickly. Keeping a pace at which you are comfortable is important to the overall process.

Also remember as you work through this new reality, there are helpful tips and tricks you can utilize to keep yourself going through the hardest parts of the commitment. For instance, you can rely on timers to remind yourself when to eat, exercise, sleep, etc. It might sound crazy but keeping a steady routine can help you keep up with your new changes. It also benefits the body and mind to have a steady routine. The tips and tricks don't stop there, though.

There are also several apps available on smartphones that you can use to track your progress. Sometimes, it takes seeing progress to really keep up that momentum. Get a fitness tracker and watch as you get closer to your goal. This everyday incentive can be a great motivator and keep you on the straight and narrow. Logging your progress can give you a sense of satisfaction that is concrete.

Finally, it might help to have an accountability partner. Let someone in on your health journey. Tell them what you are attempting to do and have them check in on your progress. Sometimes having that outside accountability can be the motivation it takes to get you out there and moving. Maybe ask if they want to be your walking or gym partner. Getting fit is always more fun when you have a buddy to walk the walk with you.

However you motivate yourself to keep up this commitment, lean into it. It's important that you make this a priority in your life and it takes a certain amount of grit to power through and do what needs to be done. You have what it takes so don't let obstacles get in your way.

Instead, view every obstacle as a new challenge and tackle it with vigor. You have what it takes to make this commitment. You just have to have the proper mindset and tools at your disposal to keep you going in spite of the difficulties you might face.

THE BOTTOM LINE

Your life is far from over. There is still so much that you add to this world. Your wisdom and unique perspective are valuable to this world so try to view your aging process through a new lens. You want to stick around for those around you, to share your gifts and passions. You want to continue doing the things that you love.

That takes a certain level of commitment. You have already started this journey by picking up this book. Keep up that momentum by putting things in place to keep you on the straight and narrow with your health. It is vital that you understand what has brought you to this point in your life. With the right motivation and the proper dedication, you can make a real change in your life so keep it up!

Of course, it's time that we start getting into how to make this vision a reality. I have already regaled you with the reasons for taking your health seriously. Now, it is time to put that into action. The next chapter will cover the role of remaining active in your life and the ways you can do that safely.

5

REMAINING ACTIVE IN YOUR TWILIGHT YEARS

As discussed in previous chapters, there are several benefits to remaining active, even in your twilight years. This cannot be stressed enough but to further drive the point home, we'll take a look at all the different ways making this change can impact you positively. It doesn't just come down to cardiovascular health and longevity. There is so much more to remaining active and living your best life.

STAYING ACTIVE, STAYING HAPPY

This may or may not surprise you but staying active goes beyond strength and endurance. It is also a great way to boost your mood. There are chemicals in the brain, which we will discuss, responsible for making us happy and they just love to come out when we are staying active. Keeping that in mind, you might find that exercising goes beyond just the physical.

Let's take a look at another study that hones in on the relationship between exercise and those happy chemicals. This study, published in *JAMA Psychiatry*, found that replacing just fifteen minutes of sitting with fifteen minutes of activity can significantly reduce the odds of depression occurring. In fact, they were able to measure the chances which were reduced by 26%.

Aside from combatting depression, activity can help you de-stress and be in a better overall mood by releasing those happy chemicals and suppressing stress hormones. This is important for so many reasons. Aside from boosting your mood, suppressing those stress hormones can keep you safe from stress-related illnesses you'd otherwise be prone to.

The great news about this is that you don't need to commit to strenuous exercise to reap the benefits. Even something as simple as taking a regular walk or doing some light yoga can help you find that peace of mind. However, it does need to be a regular thing so clear some time on your calendar every day to get that exercise in. You won't regret the decision.

Furthermore, exercising *can* be fun! Finding the right way to exercise can be key to your happiness, as you want to find something that you enjoy. For instance, some people find going to the gym boring so consider taking a Zumba class! It can be quite the workout but also greatly enjoyable. Don't let anyone tell you that staying fit has to be a dull endeavor.

We all have stress and down days but exercising can be a great way to keep yourself above water. So, pick something and stick with it. We will go over some low impact exercises later in this chapter that will be a great place to start. Just know that as you're exercising, you are not only building up your body. You are also letting those happy chemicals like serotonin and oxytocin float around that brain of yours. And that is just as important, if not more, at times.

Happier people live longer and report more feelings of purpose in their everyday life. If you want to reap these benefits, then pursuing health is a great way to start. So much of happiness is chemical reactions in our brain and learning how to train them.

With a more active lifestyle, you can expect to experience more instances of positive emotions.

STAYING ACTIVE, STAYING SHARP

Speaking of brain chemicals, I feel I should remind you about the studies that showed staying active assists in keeping your cognitive functioning from deteriorating. If you want to remain sharp into your old age, you want to start taking your fitness journey seriously. There are endless studies showing the link between these factors, giving you even more reason to get up off of that couch.

As we age, it's a reality that we have to face—our cognitive functioning begins to suffer. However, there is a way to combat this through exercising. It has been shown that exercise prevents memory loss and delays the onset of Alzheimer's symptoms in those who come down with the disease. With this knowledge, you should be taking the role of exercise in your life seriously.

For some time, researchers were not quite sure if there was a connection between exercise and brain function but recent studies have removed all doubt. One such study conducted by the Queensland Brain Institute (QBI) set out to explain this correlation. What they found was fairly cut and dry. The act of exercising increased the circulation of growth hormone (GH), adding to an increase in brain activity and increased cognitive functioning in general.

While we will be going into things like nutrition and mental wellness later in this book, it's also worth noting that there are things that you can do to keep your mind sharp. For instance, you will want to maintain good sleep hygiene, aiming for 8 hours of sleep a night. Furthermore, rely more on veggies for your calories, rather than empty carbohydrates. All of these steps have been proven to sharpen the mind and keep your brain activity at a higher level.

If you want to continue enjoying your daily Sudoku puzzle,

you'll want to keep your bodily fitness in mind. The brain is, after all, another organ in our bodies. It feels the effects of exercise the same as any organ. Primarily, the hippocampus, the portion of the brain connected to memory. By making fitness a priority, you are doing your brain a big favor.

STAYING ACTIVE, STAYING HEALTHY

I won't beat a dead horse. I have already given you plenty of examples throughout this book of how staying active impacts your bodily health. There are various studies that I've given you that point to this claim. However, it's important to understand what the best exercises are for someone who is facing the aging process.

Fitness is not a young man's game. Though there may be added concerns when working out as an older person, you can still share in the benefits of staying active. You just need to better understand your body's limitations and cultivate an exercise regime that keeps them in mind.

So, let's take a look at some low-impact exercises that are best for you. There are more options than you might expect. You just have to take your limitations into consideration as you pursue these possibilities. There is no shame in starting out slow and building up to more strenuous exercise. There is also no shame in keeping it low key. Don't feel any pressure to be a bodybuilder here. This is about remaining healthy, not about competing with others.

Water Aerobics

This might seem a bit cliche but water aerobics has actually grown in popularity in the last few years among all ages but particularly among seniors. Aside from being a lot of fun, exercising in water is also a great option for those who deal with arthritis or other types of joint pain. This is due to the buoyancy of the water putting less stress on the joints. Additionally, it eliminates the need for weights, as the water brings natural resistance.

Practices in water aerobics generally include:

- Leg lifts
- Aqua jogging
- Flutter kicking
- Standing water push-ups
- Arm curls

The benefits of water aerobics are varied but include: strength, flexibility, and balance. This is all without putting too much stress on the body. Furthermore, it is a great place to meet people as there are often group classes available at many YMCAs and local gyms with pools. This is, by far, one of the best options for seniors who want to start taking their health seriously.

Consider this option if you are worried about joint health or are looking for a place of community. I promise you won't be disappointed in the benefits this great workout can provide.

Chair Yoga

Look, I get it. You thought about yoga but you watched young people contort themselves into pretzels and decided you didn't want to risk it. However, there is a more low impact alternative that might just be perfect for you. Chair yoga has been picking up in popularity, especially for those who are worried about joint health.

Chair yoga is, simply put, exactly what it sounds like. You perform the stretching and breathing exercises inherent in yoga but from the comfort of a chair. It might sound somewhat silly but research backs up this form of exercise as still being a valid form of working out.

Like water aerobics, chair yoga is easy on the joints and helps the practitioner with benefits such as strength, mobility, balance, and flexibility. This easygoing exercise can bring you to a place where you are able to chase the kiddos around a lot easier. As an added benefit, this form of exercise has been shown to have a significant impact on mental health.

Some exercises that you can expect to practice in chair yoga are:

- Seated twist
- Overhead stretch
- Seated mountain pose
- Seated cat stretch
- Seated cow stretch

If you want an exercise that is easy on the joints and gives you more peace of mind, consider chair yoga. The benefits are innumerable and it's a great place to start for someone who might not have worked out in a while.

Resistance Band Exercises

I know what you're thinking. What exactly is resistance band training? Admittedly, it is not a well-known workout regime but the benefits of it are incredible. A resistance band is merely a large, stretchy strip of rubber or rubber tube with hand grips. Either one is very inexpensive and can be purchased both online and in sports stores. This type of exercise might seem like it's a little out of the box, but it can be a great way to stay active and build up your strength.

The best part of this exercise plan is its cost-effectiveness. The upfront cost is minimal as you merely need access to a resistance ban. Additionally, it's an ideal exercise for building your core strength, aiding in posture, mobility, and balance.

Resistance band exercises include, but are not limited to:

- Bicep curl
- Lateral raise
- Band pull apart
- Triceps press
- Leg press
- Squats

Pilates

This exercise, developed over a century ago, has become an increasingly popular form of low impact exercise. In this form of exercise, the emphasis is put on breathing, alignment, concentration, and core building. Much like yoga, it will include a mat but it also includes the use of several tools to aid the mobility of the practitioner, including yoga balls and other inflatable instruments. These aid in building up strength without the stress on the body that is included with more high impact alternatives.

Pilates is great for those who are looking for more mobility. The benefits of practicing it include balance, mobility, and increased flexibility. So if you want to get around a little easier, consider this tried and true exercise regime. In a pilates class, you can expect exercises such as:

- Leg circles
- Side circles
- Mermaid movement
- Step ups

Walking

As mentioned before, walking is an excellent and completely free way of working out. It is one of the least stressful and most accessible forms of exercising, making it a popular choice for many senior citizens. Keep in mind that your walking goal might look a bit different if you have mobility issues and feel no shame in that. For the general population, the goal sits at 10,000 steps per day. If you can aim for that, great. However, if that is something you are not able to do or you can't quite reach that goal, set your own goal! Just getting in a little bit of walking can still have a positive impact on your bodily and mental health.

The benefits of walking are astounding. Using this as your main form of exercise can bring with it tremendous benefits by strengthening muscles, increasing balance, and lowering the risk of heart disease, stroke, colon cancer, and diabetes.

There are many ways you can mix up your walking exercise to keep it fresh and enjoyable, including:

- Walking a treadmill at your local gym
- Finding a moderate trail through a park
- Training for a walk-friendly race
- Walking the perimeter of a familiar building like the mall

And you can keep yourself entertained during this activity by listening to an audiobook or uplifting music while you walk.

Body Weight Workouts

Body weight workouts are one of the best solutions to muscle loss in aging adults. Muscle loss can be devastating and affects around one-third of elderly adults. It can be extreme in its scope. It can lead to a decrease in the ability to metabolize protein, hormone imbalances, and other problems. To combat this, a simple body weight workout is optimal.

Body weight workouts are relatively low impact and have very little upfront cost, as far as materials. Some loose fitting clothes and a yoga mat are all you need to get started. These workouts can be done alone at home to a simple YouTube video or as part of a class. Some typical body weight exercises include:

- Bird dog
- Squats to chair
- Stepup
- Lying hip bridges
- Side lying circles

With the affordability and accessibility of body weight workouts, you can begin to see the benefits rather quickly. If you are among the third of aging adults who deal with muscle loss, consider this workout as part of your fitness regimen.

Dumbbell Strength Training

If you're looking to build up strength, dumbbell strength training is a great low impact exercise. The benefits of strength training, particularly for older adults, have been known to alleviate the symptoms of diabetes, osteoporosis, back pain, and even depression. It can also contribute to a higher metabolism and better glucose control. The best part? All you need is a set of dumbbells, which can be affordably purchased online or at a fitness center.

Incorporating dumbbells into your workout has innumerable benefits to your health but also aids in strengthening your core muscle group as well as your joints. You can do these workouts alone or in a group as part of a class. Some of the exercises you can expect as part of this workout include:

- Bicep curl
- Bent-over row
- Tricep extension
- Overhead press
- Front raise

Swimming

Much like water aerobics, simply swimming is a great workout that is easy on the joints and promotes a healthier lifestyle. While you will need access to a pool for this exercise, it is a great way to stay fit and active while not putting too much stress on your body. As mentioned before, the buoyancy of the water acts as natural resistance, eliminating the need for weights or other fitness equipment.

Swimming is a fun activity that also has incredible health benefits. For starters, it increases balance and stability, reducing the risk of falling. It also promotes good cardiac health and endurance. According to the Swim Strong Foundation, women can decrease the risk of cardiac conditions by 30 to 40 percent by swimming just 30 minutes per day. Likewise, men can expect to lower their risk of diabetes by 10 percent when they swim 30 minutes per day (Senionlink, 2020).

Furthermore, swimming is a great activity which provides socialization opportunities and enhanced sleep. A recent study found that regular swimming increased quality of life and sleep in self-reported analysis. So, grab your swim cap and head to the pool. Here are some types of swimming strokes you can try:

- Freestyle
- Breaststroke
- Butterfly stroke
- Backstroke

Tai Chi

Tai Chi finds its roots in martial arts developed centuries ago. The actual history is fairly hazy and mired in myth but today, the exercise is widely popular for those seeking to care for their body and mind. Because this is a full-body exercise, it provides a number of benefits that can improve your quality of life. This includes relief from arthritic pain, better balance, improved cardiovascular health, and reduced mental health struggles.

Along with pilates and yoga, tai chi has a heavy focus on breathing and flow of movement. It is all about remaining centered and balanced, both spiritually and physically. Rather than seeking to defeat an opponent, this martial art is all about bodily awareness.

Like many of the exercises listed here, the upfront cost is minimal. You might want to purchase a mat, but otherwise, it's all about your body's movement. You can opt to practice at home with videos found online or take a class at a gym or nearby park. Tai chi is an incredible workout for both your body and your mind, making it worth your time to check out.

WHAT TO AVOID

When working out in your twilight years, safety is of the utmost importance. Of course, you are not the young man or woman you once were and your body has considerations that you have to keep in mind as you look for the proper workout routine. That means that there are certain types of exercise that you will want to avoid.

While some exercises are optimal for young people to bulk up or shed weight, they can spell disaster for older adults who have problems with balance and posture. For that reason, these exercises should be avoided by anyone over the age of 65. These include:

- Squats with weights (though squats alone can be very beneficial!)
- Long distance running
- Bench press
- Leg press with weights
- Abdominal crunches
- Deadlift
- Rock climbing
- Upright row

All of these are more high impact and can put a strain on your body, most notably your joints. Keep this in mind as you exercise and remember to stay safe! Stay hydrated and keep an eye out for signs that you are overworking your body. Listen to what your body needs and if it is telling you to rest for a spell, take a hydration break.

THE BOTTOM LINE

The need for exercise cannot be denied. There are too many studies that show a direct link between staying active and lower mortality rates. Furthermore, it has a lasting impact on your mental health as well. For these reasons, you should be getting in some exercise each day, no matter what that looks like.

I have outlined some great workouts for you. Don't be afraid to try something new. There are plenty of recommendations on the list and it might take some time to find the one that works best for you. Just remember to stay away from high impact workouts that can cause undue stress on the body.

However, staying active is not the only way we should be taking care of ourselves. All factors must be considered when making a fitness plan. This includes what we are putting into our bodies. The next chapter will focus on what to eat (and what not to). So, read on for the best tips and tricks to eating healthy on a budget. I promise, you don't have to sacrifice flavor for your health, but there might be some things you can be doing better.

6

THE ROLE OF HEALTHY EATING

WHY DOES FOOD MATTER?

You might be wondering what role food plays in healthy living. After all, most of the studies I have shown you thus far have been in regards to remaining active. However, what you put into your body can have a powerful impact on your health, either positive or negative. Furthermore, as you age, what you need in terms of food can change. Your metabolism and organ function change as you age and you have to keep that in mind as you are browsing the grocery aisles.

Proper nutrition is imperative to the aging process, the other side of the equation. Eating healthy is another commitment that you must make when deciding to stay fit in your 70s. Numerous studies have been done on the relationship between healthy eating and the process of aging. The results are definitive. You can expect to see better immunity and longevity when making the right choices.

There are many things to consider when planning out a balanced diet, so let's take a look at some of them. For starters, as mentioned before, you want to make sure that you are staying hydrated. Your sense of thirst decreases as you age, so you want to stay on top of your liquid intake. To aid in this, consider picking up some fruit with high water content like melon.

Furthermore, you want to make sure that you are getting the proper amount of fiber in your diet. This ensures that things are running smoothly with your bowels, as well as lowering cholesterol levels. It can also aid in maintaining good sugar levels in your blood.

All of these things are important to consider as you walk through those grocery aisles. You want a well rounded diet that serves you, rather than acts as a detriment to your health. When you fully understand what does and doesn't need to be in your diet, you will start to make healthier long-term decisions regarding your food.

Live Longer and Stronger

Your immune system is a vital part of staying healthy. A healthy immune system means you are less likely to develop illnesses that can affect your ability to live long and strong. It has been found that nutritious eating has a direct correlation with a strengthened immune system. So when you are chowing down on that leafy green salad, remember that it's helping your body fight off illness and infection.

That's not all, however. There is also evidence linking nutritious eating to weight management, and a reduced risk of heart disease, stroke, diabetes, bone loss, and cancer. Just ensuring that you are eating a balanced diet can make a world of difference in fighting off disease and illness. Your body is a machine, working to keep you alive, and you want to fuel that machine with the best food options.

You wouldn't use cheap oil for a luxury car. You want to take care of your own hardware, as you would your transportation, if not more carefully. After all, you can always buy a new car but you are only given one body to live within throughout your lifetime. So take care of it the best way you can.

Studies also indicate that eating the right foods can give you added energy. Wholesome foods can not only make you feel and look better, but give you that added boost you need to make it through your day. This results in a boost in your self-esteem and mood. It's all connected—a full mind-body connection.

Furthermore, there is evidence that those who eat fruit, leafy greens, and foods packed with omega-3 fatty acids may be lowering their risk of Alzheimer's and improving their focus. It should be noted, however, that the best benefits in this area are seen when eating well is coupled with staying active. If you want your mind to remain sharp, make sure you are eating a balanced diet and keeping up with that fitness tracker.

WHAT TO AVOID IN THE GROCERY STORE

Let's get this out of the way first. There are foods that you should be avoiding in the grocery aisle—some which are not good at any age and some which are not suited to your particular age group. Understanding what to eliminate can be an easier place to start than with everything you want to incorporate. So let's get into it.

High Sodium Foods

We have discussed this but it is worth revisiting here. Foods high in sodium might be tempting as our taste buds dull with age. However, reaching for that salt shaker or foods high in sodium can cause problems for older adults, especially those at risk for hypertension. Whenever you are buying prepackaged food, make sure that you are reading the nutrition label for sodium content as some foods have a surprising amount. Instead of reaching for those high-sodium options, consider walking through the herb and spices aisle to add flavor to your meal.

Grapefruit

This one might surprise you. After all, I was just mentioning the benefits of adding fruits to your diet. However, this option can be a trickster. If you are taking any kind of medication, grapefruit can interfere with its efficacy. This can cause dangerous toxicity or side effects that you want to avoid. Skip over this particular citrus and opt for something like oranges or limes if you are looking to add some tanginess to your home cooked meal.

Caffeine

Yes, I know. This one hits you where it hurts. However, caffeine could be keeping you from getting a good night's sleep. Furthermore, it can even cause your heart to beat faster or more irregularly, leading to heart problems and anxiety. This is especially dangerous if you are living with any type of heart condition. Consider switching to foods that give you energy without needing that added chemical influence of caffeine.

Sugary Sodas and Sport Drinks

We just discussed caffeine but even caffeine-free sodas are chock full of sugar. Your average Coca-Cola has 39 grams of sugar in just a 12 oz serving. If you have prediabetes, these drinks can push your blood sugar into the diabetic range. Furthermore, it can cause obesity and other health issues. Try to remove sugar from your diet as much as possible, but the best place to start is with those sugary sodas. They are empty calories and don't serve you beyond that instant gratification.

Diet Sodas and Drinks

While you might be tempted to substitute your sugary beverage with a "sugar-free" alternative, these options can cause just as many issues. Recent research has shown that sugar substitutes can be linked to weight gain and a number of serious health problems. Although the calories are lower, you also might be tempted to imbibe more of these drinks, which add up over time. Best to stay away from sugar and its substitutes as much as possible.

Fatty Meats

When looking for meat to round out your meal, stay away from the fattier cuts. Though you might be tempted, these fatty cuts are loaded with saturated fats, which can wreak havoc on your body. Instead, opt for the leaner cuts and dress them up with some nice seasoning. Your body will thank you for the extra preparation. Furthermore, consider cutting out processed meats like hot dogs and bacon. Also high in saturated fats, these meats have the added detriment of being high in nitrates as well, leading to inflammation.

Soft Cheese

Though cheese is an excellent source of calcium and Vitamin D, the softer varieties can be less than ideal for older adults. This applies, in particular, to those with delicate stomachs or weakened immune systems. These varieties are rarely pasteurized and are often kept at room temperature in transit and storage. Instead of brie or goat cheese, consider going for cheddar or Colby jack cheese.

WHAT TO LOOK FOR IN THE GROCERY STORE

Now that we have eliminated some problem foods, it is time to get to the nitty gritty and talk about what will best serve you as you age. There are certain foods that will aid in living a healthier, more balanced life. Coupled with the right exercise routine, they can add years to your life and energy to your day. Look for these foods in the grocery aisles next time you go shopping! It can make all the difference!

Fruits and Vegetables

It goes without saying that one of the healthiest things you can do for your diet is to start incorporating more fresh fruit and veggies. Fruit is a great way to satisfy that sweet tooth without reaching for the sugar. However, break out of the rut of apples and bananas and look for something a bit more rich in color such as berries and melons.You will want to aim for 2-3 servings of fruit per day. As for vegetables, you want to look for the variety that are rich in antioxidants such as dark leafy greens. Think spinach, kale, and broccoli. Also look at colorful veggies such as squash or carrots. And don't think that this needs to be a chore. Saute some of those vegetables in olive oil and some seasoning for a delicious treat. Much like fruits, you want to aim for 2-3 servings of vegetables a day.

When looking for fruits and veggies, it is preferable to buy fresh. Some of the nutrients are lost in the freezing process. However, if you find that you only have time to prepare vegetables that are frozen, they are better than forgoing them altogether. Still, consider taking some extra time in the kitchen to prepare these fresh vegetables and all the nutrients they can provide you.

Calcium-Rich Foods

As you age, your bones lose density. It is just one of the realities of growing older. To combat this, you want to make sure that you have a good amount of calcium in your diet. This can aid in fighting osteoporosis and bone fractures. You just have to make sure that you are eating the right foods such as milk, yogurt, and cheese. Alternatively, if you want a dairy-free source, you can find it in tofu, broccoli, almonds, and kale. In order to keep those bones nice and strong, make sure you are incorporating these foods into your diet.

Varied Proteins

As you age, you will find that eating an adequate amount of protein can improve your mood, boost your stress response, and even help you think more clearly. You want to aim for variety to make sure that you are getting the best benefits from your protein source. Some great foods to consider when picking a protein source include: fish (great source of omega-3 as well!), lean poultry, beans, peas, and nuts. Try to stay away from processed meats when picking a protein, as mentioned above. The saturated fats and nitrates can lead to inflammation and other health problems. Instead, stick to whole proteins.

Foods Rich in B Vitamins

For some energy to get you through your day, you might also want to consider seeking out foods that are rich in B vitamins. B12 and B6 are great for that added boost, as well as promoting the generation of healthy cells in the body. The great thing about these vitamins is that they can be found in a variety of foods. Salmon, for instance, is a great source. You can also add to the list: leafy greens, eggs, milk, legumes, and beef.

Foods Rich in Vitamin C

Let's face it. The hardest thing to deal with as we age is coming down with some kind of bug. It can drain our energy and leave us feeling weak. That's why it is important to make sure that your immune system is properly bolstered by the right vitamins. Vitamin C is a great vitamin to ensure that your immune system has a fighting chance. Foods that include high quantities of Vitamin C are: citrus fruits (remember to stay away from grapefruit, though), peppers, strawberries, broccoli, and potatoes.

PERFECT MEALS FOR A WELL BALANCED DIET

I've given you a variety of options to start your healthy eating kick. However, it is important to understand how to combine these dos and don'ts into a healthy meal that you can enjoy. That's where meal prep comes in. The best way to make sure that you are staying on the straight and narrow with your eating habits is to commit to planning out your meals. And make sure they are delicious!

The key is balance. You want a little bit of everything on your plate—the right vitamins, protein, calcium, etc. If you can find a way to have all of these on the same plate, you're on the right track. So, let's take a look at what this actually looks like in action.

First, make sure that you have your protein. We discussed the proper types of protein to include in your meal. Stay away from processed meat and fatty cuts. Fish is a great option for a protein so perhaps planning to have something like salmon or tuna a few times a week could be something you might incorporate. Secondly, make sure you are including those veggies, preferably something rich in vitamins and antioxidants. Finally, make sure there *are* some carbs on your plate, but seek out carbs that give some added benefits like potatoes, rather than most breads, which can amount to empty calories.

To give you an idea of what this can look like day to day, I've outlined a simple weeklong meal plan. This can be altered to your personal taste but I wanted to show you exactly what a well-balanced meal plan would be for someone in your age category. Keep in mind, there might be nutritional restrictions that you have in place that I am not aware of so this is hardly a "one-size-fits-all" meal plan. It is just a place from which you can begin.

Day One

Breakfast: Poached egg on two slices of whole wheat toast
Morning snack: 1 cup blueberries
Lunch: One serving of Loaded Black Bean Nacho Soup
Afternoon snack: One medium-sized orange
Dinner: Seared salmon with green beans, and one baked red potato

Day Two

Breakfast: Bran cereal with skim milk and blueberries
Morning snack: An apple with nut butter
Lunch: Strawberry and spinach salad with light dressing
Afternoon snack: An orange or a handful of raspberries
Dinner: Charred shrimp pesto pasta

Day Three

Breakfast: Greek yogurt with blueberries, almonds, and a honey drizzle
Morning snack: A cup of raspberries
Lunch: Kale salad with tuna and almonds
Afternoon Snack: Apple with cheddar cheese
Dinner: Sweet potato and peanut soup, whole wheat bread

Day Four

Breakfast: Avocado on whole grain toast with scrambled egg, ½ cup of blueberries
Morning snack: Greek yogurt and an apple
Lunch: Lentil soup, whole wheat roll
Afternoon snack: Bell peppers with hummus
Dinner: Sweet potato stuffed with shredded salmon, side of peas

Day Five

Breakfast: Two slices of whole wheat toast with sunflower butter spread, honey, and banana
Morning snack: Pear with cheddar cheese
Lunch: Home-made carrot and parsnip soup, whole wheat roll
Afternoon snack: Carrot sticks with hummus
Dinner: Chicken and vegetable traybake

Day Six

Breakfast: Whole wheat toast with low-fat cream cheese
Morning snack: Apple with nut butter
Lunch: Jacket potato with baked beans (look out for a brand without added sugar and salt), Kale salad
Afternoon snack: Handful of almonds
Dinner: Cottage pie with peas and carrots (use lean meat when making)

Day Seven

Breakfast: Greek yogurt with granola and berries
Morning snack: Medium orange
Lunch: Sweet potato, kale, and peanut salad with light dressing
Afternoon snack: Handful of dry-roasted almonds
Dinner: Lentil stew, whole wheat roll

This meal plan is not meant to be set in stone but merely a guide toward what foods you should gravitate to for a well-balanced diet. You can find helpful recipes for meal prep on sites like Eating Well and The Geriatric Dietician. The important thing to remember is that everyone is different and has different dietary needs, especially as we age. Speak with your doctor before planning out your meals and ask them if there are any further considerations you need to keep in mind.

Try to follow these meal ideas but don't feel that you are bound by them. There is also personal taste to consider. You want to make sure that you are eating foods that you also *enjoy* to ensure that you continue with your nutritional diet plan. If you aren't a fan of the food you are eating, odds are that you won't stick with the program and fall off the wagon. So, if certain things need to be adjusted, feel free to do so. Just make sure you keep the nutritional value of your substitutes in mind.

THE BOTTOM LINE

Eating the right foods can seem daunting at first. However, with the knowledge I have provided in this chapter, you are more equipped to make the correct decisions when it comes to grocery shopping. Furthermore, planning out your meals is a great way to make things less daunting and to keep you from eating according to your cravings. Things will begin to come more easily as you get used to the process of nutritional eating. As a bonus, you will begin to look and feel better.

Exercising is great but it needs to work in tandem with healthy eating choices. You need the proper fuel to get out there and stay active. It is imperative to your health that you start making the right decisions about your eating as working with your body's nutritional needs is beneficial to its functioning.

There are a variety of nutrients and vitamins vital to a body's proper functioning. Within this chapter, we have covered a great many of them. Keeping these in mind as you peruse the grocery aisles will help you make the right decisions.

Of course, there are also other ways to ensure that you are getting the vitamins you need as you age. Supplements have grown in popularity in recent years and their benefits can be fantastic. However, there are considerations that you will want to keep in mind as you shop for just the right supplement. We will cover that in the next chapter.

7

TO SUPPLEMENT OR NOT?

Supplements are a great resource for those who struggle to get the proper amount of vitamins and nutrients from their average diet. However, it is important to consider each supplement for its benefits and drawbacks. Not every supplement on the market is equal and not all of them will serve you. A practical guide to modern supplements will help you steer through the market and select what will serve you best.

SUPPLEMENTS AND WHAT THEY DO

Before we get into brass tacks about what supplements can do for you, it's important to understand what they are and their function in your health journey. Simply put, supplements are capsules, powders, pills, or even gummies that contain vital vitamins, minerals, and enzymes for healthy living. While you should not rely on supplements in place of healthy eating, they can give you an added boost if you are lacking in any certain area.

The idea of these supplements is just that—to "supplement" healthy eating and exercise. They should not be used in place of either but rather in tandem. It should bridge the gap of any dietary deficiencies you might be experiencing. Furthermore, some people have a harder time absorbing certain nutrients and might actually *need* to supplement those vitamins. For instance, if you don't spend much time outdoors, it can be hard to get enough Vitamin D from just food. Therefore, a supplement might be your best option, given the circumstances.

However, not all supplements are created equal and it's important to keep certain things in mind as you shop around for the best ones. Numerous supplements exist and quite often, they can claim unfounded benefits, as they are not approved for such usage. Although a supplement might seem harmless, keep these things in mind.

1. There is very little oversight and regulation regarding supplements, and they are treated differently than food and medications. They do not need to prove their safety prior to being put on the market and it's only after they reach the shelves that FDA will intervene. Make sure you are buying from a reputable brand.

2. Just because something is "natural," it doesn't necessarily mean that it's good or safe for you to use. What worked for your neighbor might not be what you specifically need. Keep in mind where you are getting your information from and seek out reputable sources before taking any supplements.

3. Finally, even though these are general vitamins and minerals that you might need, there is still a possibility of interactions with medication. Do not take any supplements before first discussing them with your doctor, who can help you navigate safely through the market.

Don't let this scare you away from supplements as ones that are produced under good manufacturing practices can still be beneficial to your overall health. Just remain cautious as you begin this journey. You want to make sure that you are bolstering your health, rather than jeopardizing it. Keep your doctor appraised of all supplements you are thinking of taking and discuss your options. Also, asking for their suggestions on brands is a great idea.

There are a number of supplements on the market that are targeted toward the elderly population but I have compiled a list of some of the most helpful supplements and what they provide for your health. It can help to have a starting point before wading into the waters. Frankly, the variety on the shelves can be overwhelming.

Calcium

Calcium is undoubtedly one of the most important supplements I can suggest to you. It works alongside Vitamin D to ensure that your bones are remaining strong. This is especially important as you age and lose bone density. It can be hard to keep up with the necessary calcium intake requirements for your body, so adding this to supplement your levels can be a great idea.

Vitamin D

It is widely known that most people are deficient in Vitamin D. It can be hard for those of us who don't spend much time outdoors to absorb the proper amount of the vital vitamin. You can find it in foods like citrus and vitamin-D fortified milk but relying on diet alone can often not give us the correct levels we need. Vitamin D is linked to energy, your immune system, and bone strength. With the importance linked to so many bodily systems, it is imperative that you make sure your levels are good. Check with your doctor about getting a blood test done before taking this, to see if you are, in fact, deficient and talk to them about best options for moving forward.

Vitamin B12

Vitamin B12 is a great vitamin to keep your red blood cells and nerves healthy. This can aid in overall health but also is great for any type of disorders that affect those areas of the body. While older adults don't necessarily need more of this vitamin than others, it has been found that they have a harder time absorbing it through food. That is why many doctors recommend older adults taking a supplement for B12 to make sure that they are on track with their levels. Have a discussion with your doctor about whether this supplement is right for you.

Vitamin B6

This nifty supplement is great for keeping your blood cell count at a healthy level. While B vitamins can be found in abundance in many healthy foods like chicken and potatoes, you might still need to supplement your intake. As an added bonus, B vitamins are great for energy so if you are looking for a little boost in your day, this can be a great option for you.

Folic Acid

Also known as vitamin B9, folic acid is another great vitamin that can benefit an aging adult (or really anyone). It works particularly well with memory, preventing memory loss in those over the age of 60. Not only that but it aids in converting carbohydrates to energy. Another great vitamin to give you the boost that you might need to get you through your day, while also working to keep your mind sharp. If you wish to find this vitamin in your food, you can find it in broccoli, brussel sprouts, and spinach. However, supplements are designed to ensure that you are getting the right dosage for your specific needs.

Acetyl-L-Carnitine (ALCAR)

This one sure is a mouthful but believe it or not, it is one of my most highly recommended supplements for those on the older age of the spectrum. This supplement is absolutely crucial to the functioning of your mitochondria. You might remember from your school days that the mitochondria are a part of the cell that powers it. This is good news, as recent studies have shown that this supplement might offer relief from age-related fatigue and cognitive decline. The NIH Office of Dietary Supplements has come out to say that this supplement may very well help those who experience mild cognitive impairment or the beginning stages of Alzheimer's Disease.

Omega Fatty Acids

Omega-3 fatty acids and omega-6 fatty acids greatly impact your overall health. Research shows that omega fatty acids reduce pain and other symptoms of rheumatoid arthritis, and macular degeneration that leads to loss of vision or vision weakness. Furthermore, they give you added energy that can get you through the day. The best ways to get omega fatty acids into your diet would be through fish or walnuts. However, taking a supplement is a great way to make sure that you are getting enough of those healthy fats to feel the full benefits.

Coenzyme Q10

Also known at CoQ10, this supplement is actually an antioxidant that is naturally produced in the liver. However, as we age, our livers become less effective at producing it and it can be very difficult to find it through food sources. That is why this is a great supplement to add to your daily routine as you age. Low levels of CoQ10 have been associated with heart disease, especially in those in their twilight years. The best way to make sure your levels are where they should be is to take a trusted supplement. Talk to your doctor about this possibility.

Multivitamin

There has been some back and forth on the efficacy of multivitamins. Though they preach incredible benefits, the same benefits can also be found in eating right and exercising. However, there are often still vitamin deficiencies in our diet, especially as we age, and a multivitamin can cover a lot of bases. Look for one that is specifically geared towards older adults as they will include vitamins that tend to decline with age. Speak to your doctor about the best choice of multivitamin.

Glucosamine

Do you experience joint pain? As our bodies age, the cartilage wears down and arthritis can cause significant pain in our joints. If this is something you struggle with, I would recommend adding glucosamine to your regimen. Though I must admit a bias, as I take it for joint pain, I can also attest to its efficacy. Glucosamine works by keeping up the health of your cartilage, the rubbery tissue that connects your bones at the joint. By supporting this part of your body, there is less pain around the joint. Talk to your doctor if this seems like something you would benefit from.

SHOULD YOU BE TAKING THEM?

Unlike diet and exercise, there is some disagreement on whether taking supplements is necessary or beneficial to the individual user. As mentioned before, not all supplements are created equal, and first and foremost, you want to make sure you are purchasing supplements from a reputable source. Look up reviews online and be diligent about where you are getting your information. Make sure that the sites from which you get your information comes from reputable professionals such as doctors, researchers, or dieticians.

Also, as mentioned before, you want to make sure that you are keeping your doctor apprised of any supplements you are considering. Your doc can safely steer you towards the best brands *and* navigate through what is actually needed. Furthermore, they can explain any interactions that these supplements might have with your existing medications. Not everything is safe simply because it is "natural." Everything is a chemical compound that can cause serious interactions if not taken safely and in the right dosages.

While taking supplements is a great way to make up for any deficits in your diet, it is not a substitute for eating right and exercising. They are merely there to add to what you are already doing. So don't rely on popping a multivitamin for your health. This can be disappointing, as taking a simple capsule sounds so much easier but truly, you will experience much more improvement when you use them in tandem with your already healthy lifestyle.

If you begin taking a supplement and start noticing any unfortunate side effects, stop taking the supplement right away and give your doctor a call. Either you are reacting poorly to the compound (due to personal aversions or poor manufacturing). First and foremost, you want to be safe while taking these supplements which means keeping track of your reactions to them.

In the end, I cannot tell you whether supplements are for you or not. That is only a decision that you can make in partnership with your doctor. I can only provide you with the information to go into that appointment informed and ready to make the call. It is my hope that you feel more prepared to make those decisions going forward.

THE BOTTOM LINE

Supplements can be a great way to bridge the gap between the nutrients you're taking in and what you still need. This goes doubly for nutrients that your aging body has a hard time producing or absorbing. However, safety must always come first and it's imperative that you go about taking these supplements the right way. Seek out reputable sources for your supplements, talk to your doctor, and always trust what your body is trying to tell you.

If you feel that supplements could help you on your health journey, great! But know that the exact benefits can differ from person to person. What worked for someone else might not be the miracle supplement you were hoping for. Furthermore, if you decide not to use supplements, you will want to make sure that your diet is targeting the particular nutrients you desperately need. Refer back to chapter five when it comes to eating a healthy balanced diet.

Now that we have talked about the great benefits of staying physically fit, we should also discuss the importance of mental wellbeing. There are numerous studies that show that a focus on mental health can also have added benefits to your physical health. It is all tied in together. While you're taking care of your body, let's take a look at what you need to do to take care of your mind.

8

MENTAL WELL-BEING

Mental health has been a topic of much discussion over the past decade. More and more, medical professionals are discovering links between your mental well-being and your physical health. But more than that, it is important to take care of your mental health because it *is* a part of your overall health. Aging can be a difficult process and now, more than ever, you want to make sure that you are taking care of yourself.

Now, I know what you are thinking. However, self-care isn't all about bath bombs and chocolates. It is about creating a life for yourself that you *don't* need to constantly escape from. To set yourself up for success, you might have to do some hard work but don't worry. I will walk you through some of the basics to get you started.

WHY MENTAL HEALTH IS IMPORTANT AS YOU AGE

The fact of the matter is, growing old can be hard on the body *and* mind. As you go through the aging process, you are actually more prone to develop mental health issues such as depression. This can occur due to changes in your body or changes in your lifestyle. Whatever the reason, it is important to notice the signs of a mental health issue early and take them seriously. Depression has been linked to an increased risk of conditions such as diabetes, heart disease, and stroke. Some signs that you might be experiencing depression are:

- Noticable changes in mood, energy levels, and appetite
- Feeling emotionally flat or having a hard time feeling positive emotions
- Feeling restless and on edge
- Difficulty concentrating
- Increased worry or feelings of stress
- Sadness or hopelessness
- Suicidal thoughts
- Anger, irritability, and increased aggression
- Obsessive thinking or compulsive behavior

While these are not sure fire ways to diagnose depression, they can point to a mental health problem that should be seen to by a doctor. Talk to your general practitioner if you feel that you might be depressed and talk through the options with them. While exercise and diet can greatly improve mood, there are also other options to consider like medication or therapy.

However, even if you aren't clinically depressed, it is still important to safeguard your mental wellbeing. Having a well-balanced emotional state is just as important as having a strong, healthy body. Taking care of both your body *and* mind is important. Why? Because your mental health affects your physical health and vice versa. Taking care of yourself, body and mind is imperative for a well-lived life.

There are special considerations regarding aging, when talking about mental health. An older adult is likely to have the same stressors as those from younger demographics. However, they are more frequently plagued with stressors like lack of mobility, chronic pain, and other health problems. These stressors can exert a nasty toll so it's imperative that you take the steps necessary to deal with your mental health, whatever state it might currently be in.

Yes, that's right. It's important that you make your mental health a priority, even when things are going well. The fact is, life will not always be going well, and you should be prepared for those moments when things are especially difficult. This chapter seeks to guide you through common mental health challenges and the practices that will help you overcome them.

WHAT THE STUDIES HAVE TO SAY

As the human race has begun to live longer and longer, more studies have been done regarding the mental health of the elderly. The results are astounding and bring to light the importance of maintaining proper mental hygiene while aging. According to these studies, as many as 20 percent of older adults and up to 37 percent of those living in assisted living facilities suffer from depression (U.S. Department of Health and Human Services 2001).

Despite these harrowing statistics, less than three percent of older adults report seeing a mental health professional to address these problems. That is not only concerning, but it can also be disastrous. If you believe that you are experiencing symptoms of depression, make sure you are discussing it with your doctor and figuring out your options.

Of course, there are reasons that so many fail to seek help. Among these reasons are lack of proper resources and lack of properly trained mental health professionals who cater specifically to those in the later stages of life. This can make it difficult to seek out and acquire the help needed to make it through these challenges.

Mental health isn't just about the mind, though it starts there. Studies have found direct connections between declining mental health and a decline in overall health. Mental health issues like depression have been linked to an increase in heart disease, strokes, diabetes, and several other health problems.

To avoid falling into this cycle, you must take an active approach. You want to make sure that you are taking the steps necessary to take care of your mental health *now*, before it becomes an issue down the line. Even if you aren't currently suffering from a mental disorder, there are things you can do to ensure that your state of mind stays well balanced.

Some of these practices might seem a little out there, but I swear by them when it comes to tending to your mental health. Committing yourself to these practices can be a change of pace but coupling them with exercising and eating right can make all the difference in your overall health. Treat this as a prescription—for your mind!

SIMPLE PRACTICES FOR MINDFUL AND FULFILLED LIVING

I have thrown a lot of information at you in this book and I hope that you have persisted to this point. This is where a real transformation occurs. Taking control of your mental health can directly influence your success in the other areas of this book. Start making it a priority and listen to what the experts have to say about mental health and seniors.

You might be thinking that this chapter isn't for you. However, we all have emotional baggage and stressors that can cause us to worry and feel down. Taking the proper steps toward self-care is imperative when dealing with these issues. But what exactly does self- care look like, you might ask?

Self-care has become a bit of a buzzy phrase in recent years. It's been discussed ad nauseum on social media, and I feel that a lot of the dialogue doesn't quite hit the mark. Self-care isn't always about eating comfort food in your pajamas. A lot of times, it is hard work to maintain your emotional and spiritual wellbeing. It is about taking the steps you need to in order to live a life where you feel fulfilled.

So, where do you start? Honestly, implementing exercise and a nutritional diet is a great place to start so you're already in a good position to tackle these practices. However, there is more to mental health than taking care of your physical body. You also should be doing things that nourish your mind and heart.

There are many ways you can do this so let's look at some of the simple ones first:

Take a Hike! (Or Walk)

This was noted in the earlier chapter but going on walks is a type of exercise that can nourish your mind as well as your body. Take some time out in nature and listen to the sounds around you. Perhaps carry a guide book to identify birds as you hike along a woodsy trail. Or you can take an easy path around a pond and watch how the sun reflects off the water. Taking in the fresh air and the nature around you is a great way to make you feel more connected with life and get those happy chemicals firing. What's more, you can accompany your walk with an enriching audiobook or uplifting music to really set the mood for a good day. Taking a walk can make a huge difference in your mental wellbeing.

Stay Connected

This particular topic will be covered more in-depth in the next chapter but it bears acknowledgment here. This really should go without saying, but we are a social species. We are designed to rely on each other. So, community is an important part of anyone's life. The genuine connections you make with other people can keep your mood up and your mind sharp as you age. If you don't have a current community, consider signing up for a class that you can take at a local community center with like minded individuals—a book club, a writing class, or a support group. Likewise, you can sign up for group exercise classes and make friends and connections there. Having people in your life who care about you and for whom you care is vitally important to mental wellness as you age.

Pick Up a New Hobby

What are you passionate about? What sparks joy in your heart? Whatever popped into your head, see if there is a hobby that will let you enjoy that passion. If you're a nature nut, look into bird watching or hiking. If you love putting things together with your hands, consider woodworking or assembling model kits. There are a good number of hobbies accessible to older adults that might interest you—knitting, painting, writing. Whatever makes you feel alive, go out and do it as much as you can. This is the time to mark things off your bucket list, so if you ever wanted to write a book, pick up that pen (or likely, laptop) and get to it! These passions will be a driving force to keep you going.

Volunteering

My favorite thing about having more time for myself these days is that I've been able to donate some of it to causes I believe in. If you have a cause you are passionate about, consider volunteering your time. There are many animal shelters looking for volunteers to socialize with the animals. Likewise, you could volunteer for charities that bless children in hospitals with toys, or spread the word about a cause that means a lot to you. There are different avenues for finding volunteer opportunities from checking out your local library newsletter to checking the bulletin board at your local church or community center. However you are able to volunteer, it's a great way to share your passion and skills with the world and give you purpose.

Caring for a Pet

I want to preface this one by stating that pet ownership might not be a possibility for all older adults. There are numerous obstacles to owning a pet such as housing rules, cost, and general mobility. However, if you are able to, caring for a pet is a great way to put some meaning and purpose into your day. Furthermore, you get to enjoy the love and cuddles from your furry friend, which has been shown to decrease loneliness as well as your blood pressure! If you've been thinking about getting a pup or a cat, maybe this is your sign it is time to go for it. You will find your life enriched and uplifted by their presence.

Surround Yourself With What You Love

I know that this one gets talked about a bit dismissively and for good reason—it can be taken too far. People drain their bank account by tapping "add to cart" too much. But there can be a healthy balance. Maybe treat yourself to your favorite meal at your favorite restaurant once a month. Or every now and then, buy *yourself* some flowers. Treat yourself in little ways as an act of self-love. They can make all the difference when you are having a rough time. Sprinkle some joy here and there and you will find that life is more worth living. It is just as important to show yourself love as it is to show yourself discipline. Just walk the line with care.

Maintain Good Sleep Hygiene

This is another one that should go without saying but having a good sleep schedule is imperative to physical *and* mental wellness. Try to sleep for an average of 7-9 hours a night and keep your sleeping routine fairly regular. A scattered sleep schedule can wreak havoc on your body and mood. Furthermore, having a steady routine in general can aid you in getting a good night's rest on a regular basis. Try to eat and workout at the same time every day to ensure that your body knows when it is time to wind down for the evening. Create a ritual to wind down. Perhaps that looks like making a cup of tea and watching a relaxing TV show. Maybe it is cuddling up with a book. Whatever you choose as your nighttime ritual, stick to it and it will ease you into sleep with much more efficacy.

Practice Mindfulness

Mindfulness is about remaining in the present moment. It's about forgetting the to-do lists and plans for one moment to really revel in *now*. Two practices that can help you maintain this balance are yoga and meditation. We already discussed yoga, which puts the focus on breath, movement, and spiritual alignment. Meditation is another alternative for those looking for a less active approach to their mindfulness. There are many apps you can download or free audiobook meditations available that can guide you through the steps toward mindfulness.

Furthermore, there are small practices you can put into place for when you are feeling stressed and need to remain grounded.

For starters, you can do what is called a body scan. A body scan is when you mentally take note of the sensations in your body, working your way down from your head all the way to your feet. Letting yourself experience and acknowledge those sensations can keep you grounded and steady when stressors might be knocking at your door.

Another one of my favorite practices is the 5-4-3-2-1 technique. This can be a self-soothing tactic for when you are stressed or upset. The basis of the practice is simple. Hone in on five things you can see, four things you can hear, three things you can feel, two things you can smell, and one thing you can taste. No matter where you are, this is a technique you can employ to ground yourself and stay present in the moment. Even if you are not in active distress, it helps to practice these mindfulness rituals so that they come easier as life gets crazy.

Finally, as mentioned before regarding yoga, paying attention to your breathing can bring grounding and stillness to any moment. One of my favorite breathing practices is called "square breathing." This technique is simple and effective to calm down nerves or anxiety. You simply inhale through your nose for four seconds, hold the breath for four seconds, and exhale for—you guessed it—four seconds. This helps regulate your body's oxygen flow and can bring some stillness to an anxiety-inducing moment.

Mindful coloring and drawing is also another way to stay present while creatively expressing yourself. Instead of paying close attention to the shapes in the coloring book or what you're attempting to draw, hone in one the sensation of the pencil rubbing against the paper. Be mindful of how your hand works with the artistic implement to create something.

These mindfulness practices are all great ways to ground yourself and ward off worry. However, they are also great for decreasing the risk of anxiety and depression. You are at a time in your life when you are particularly susceptible to these ailments so keep tabs on your mindfulness and see what you can do to bring your mind into the present with you.

Practice Self-Soothing

Self-soothing and grounding often get used interchangeably but they are actually quite different in nature. While mindfulness demands that your mind stay present in the moment, self-soothing can have a broader scope. Whatever soothes you from reading a book to lighting a special candle can bring peace to your soul and help you through stress. Learning how to self-regulate your stresses can be difficult but when you have habits that you automatically turn to in times of high stress, then you can begin learning how to do so slowly. Keep your coping skills around you and you will find that you can face your anxieties with more ease.

Have a Good Routine

I have mentioned this a few times before it bears repeating here. One of the best ways to create a sound mind is to stick to a routine. I know that I have thrown a lot of new things at you so this might feel dichotomous. However, when it comes to your day-to-day activities, it is best to attempt a schedule. Try doing the same things around the same time every day. Our bodies and minds thrive on routine and you might find that your sleep and energy levels are better for it. If at first you struggle to maintain a routine, try setting alarms for yourself. I know they have been a lifesaver for me at times. Furthermore, assure that you are taking any medications at the same time every day. Their efficacy often depends on this. All around, having a good routine is good for the mind, body, and soul. Keep to a schedule and you might see great improvements in all of the above.

THE BOTTOM LINE

Your mental well-being is as important as the wellbeing of your body. This is because the two are intertwined. Neglecting one of these areas will not serve you in the other. Due to the increase in depression and anxiety rates among seniors, it is vitally important that you make your mental health a priority. It can decrease your risk of loneliness and low moods, while also lowering your risk for heart disease and stroke.

There are a number of great ways to cater to your mental health. I have listed out several for you but there are innumerable resources available for those seeking to improve their mental health in their twilight years. Consider downloading a mood tracker app and a meditation app on your phone. Download some helpful audiobooks to listen to on your walks.

Most of all, mental wellness is not a one size fits all prescription. You will have to find what works for you. While some things are necessary to all humans—community and a good sleep routine —others should be more tailored to the individual. Take what works for you and leave the rest.

You don't want to become a statistic. However, if you do find yourself experiencing symptoms of depression and anxiety, common disorders in older adults, reach out to your health care provider. They should be able to connect you with resources to see to your mental health. Whether that is evaluating medications or seeking out therapy, there is a way out of the darkness.

Of course, one of the best ways I have found to combat the darkness is to remain connected to fellow human beings. We are a social species and it's important that we make connection a priority in our lives. The next chapter will give you some practical steps on how to stay connected with friends and family. (Plus make new ones!)

9

STAYING CONNECTED

While I have touched on this several times throughout this book, I felt like it deserved its own chapter. As a species, we were designed to live as a pack. We are social creatures and that plays a huge part in our overall health. In staying connected, we have a meaning behind our health journey. We find purpose in the lives of others.

WHY CONNECTION IS SO IMPORTANT

You might be asking why connection is so important, and that's a fair question. We live in a world where we are more connected than ever, yet somehow are more lonely than we ever have been before. It's a dichotomy that leaves us wanting for something. It is no surprise that we are happier when we are connected with others. However, there are other benefits to staying looped in that you might not even realize. Some of these incredible health benefits include:

- Disease prevention
- Increased length of life
- Fewer physical health problems
- Improved cognitive function
- Sense of belonging
- Better self-esteem
- Maintained purpose of life

As you can see, there are a great many benefits to staying connected to your fellow man, both physical and otherwise. However, you don't have to take my word for it. Studies have been conducted to prove these claims. Let's start with disease prevention. This one, after all, might seem somewhat surprising. The truth, though, is that connectedness can stave off illness.

For over fifty years, researchers have focused on the role of community and a sense of belonging in human health. As far back as the 60sn and 70s, researchers followed Alameda County residents, attempting to measure the impact of "community" on health. Community was measured by religious affiliations, volunteering, and the number of friends and acquaintances. This study showed remarkable results—those with a strong sense of community experienced notably lower rates of disease and tended to live longer.

Furthermore, community isn't just about avoiding disease. There is something rather special about a sense of belonging. It nourishes the mind in a way that can keep you in a healthier place, both physically and emotionally. Those who are deeply connected to a community also don't question their spiritual beliefs and remain firm in them, giving them purpose.

Loneliness is a cancer that can deeply affect those who feel it. When you remain connected with a community, you can combat that loneliness with true belonging. There are ways that you can remain connected to those around you, even if right now, you are feeling that loneliness. You just need to find your community. The next section will go over some great ways that you can achieve that.

Don't be a wallflower. Get out there and make some new friends, or reconnect with old ones. It is about so much more than your Facebook friends list. It is about your health both emotional and physical.

HOW TO STAY CONNECTED

Okay, so you understand the need for community but you aren't entirely sure how to find it. You have made it this far on your own but now you yearn for more. There are some great ways to stay connected. You just have to put in the effort. This isn't just about loneliness. This has been proven to improve your health. So, without further ado, here are some great ideas that can keep you within a community.

Start Volunteering

This was mentioned in the chapter on mental health and there's a reason for that. It is not only a way to find purpose, but to find other like-minded individuals. When you volunteer in groups, you find connectedness with others. You are bonded together by a common goal and passion. You can look into volunteering at the local hospital or at the library—anywhere you might find some meaningful relationships while also making a difference.

Take a Fitness Class

To go along with the theme of this book, one of the greatest ways to meet new people is to join a fitness class! There are several options available to you through local gyms and community centers. You can try a yoga class or a swimming class. You are getting in a good workout while also getting to know others who are starting that same journey. It can be incredibly beneficial to you on several levels.

Give Someone a Call

With the world the way it is, you might find yourself far fro0m family and friends. That doesn't mean you have to stay distant. Technology has come a long way to keep us connected. If you want to reach out to a friend or family member from across the country, do it! With FaceTime, you can even see their smiling faces. Staying connected doesn't have to be complicated. Just pick up that phone and reach out to a loved one. I'm sure they would love to hear from you.

Consider making this a regular appointment. Just like you would schedule lunch dates, set up a time every week when you call and talk for a time with your loved one. It gives you something to look forward to and keeps you connected with someone you care about. Take advantage of today's incredible technology and stay in contact with those far away.

Stay Involved With Your Church

This one might not be for everybody. I am fully aware that not everyone is religious so if this one doesn't speak to you, feel free to skip it. However, for those who follow a particular faith, staying active in the church can be a great way to maintain community while also serving a higher purpose. Consider volunteering for a committee or attending regular church functions. Bring a casserole to the potluck or volunteer to teach Sunday school. There are innumerable ways to stay active in your church and stay connected with your community. Ask around if there is a Bible study you can join.

You will be surrounded by like-minded individuals who want to see you grow in your faith, and that is a beautiful thing.

Pursue a Group Hobby

If you have a hobby that you would like to pursue, see if there are any classes that cater to a group setting. There are plenty of clubs and groups you can join through community centers and libraries. For instance, there might be a hiking group or a woodworking class you can take. Whatever the hobby, there is likely a class or group that you can join up with to fully pursue your passion.

This one is great for two reasons. For starters, it connects you with like minded individuals who can encourage you as you pursue your passions. Secondly, it gives you an opportunity to do something that brings you joy. Give this option a try if you're looking for ways to get out of the house and connected with others.

Befriend Your Neighbors

This one I saved for last because it can be a difficult task. Putting yourself out there is difficult but it helps to get to know your neighbors as you age. You will have a built-in support system close to home. Try taking a casserole over to your neighbor's place and introduce yourself. Invite them over for a game night or whatever floats your boat. Do your best to engage in the community around you. This can leave you feeling safer and less lonely.

THE BY-PRODUCTS OF CONNECTIVITY

While connectedness can be great for our health, both mental and physical, it also has a lot of great by-products that often get forgotten in health books like this. Sure, you are experiencing more of those happy chemicals and you are less prone to disease. However, that's not all that you can expect to find when remaining more connected to your community.

You will find a new sense of drive. When you are around other like-minded individuals, you tend to burn a fire under each other. Take, for instance, participating in a class for a new hobby. That class can push you further than pursuing that hobby on your own. The feedback and challenge of keeping up with your peers can keep you on your toes.

You will also find that loneliness finds you left often. Sure, we all get lonely from time to time. However, it's a real problem for those who are in their twilight years. Due to family moving away and losing friends, elder adults can find that loneliness is an ever present companion. However, with more connection to those around them, it keeps that particular demon at bay.

Furthermore, you will find inspiration in the everyday more often. And it is something that you will be able to pass on. When it comes to activities like volunteering, you are more in tune with the world around you and you will start to notice incredible moments happening right before your eyes. It's easy to get lost in the dark news cycle and lose sight of the goodness in humanity. However, by remaining connected to it on a deep, personal level, you can find yourself seeing it more and more.

THE BOTTOM LINE

The importance of community cannot be understated. This goes doubly for those who are entering their twilight years. It doesn't just stave off the loneliness but actually increases your ability to fend off disease. The research is there to support so you have no reason to seclude yourself when there is a beautiful community waiting to get to know you.

There are many options available to you when it comes to

community engagement. From volunteering in your community to remaining active in your church, you have options. You just have to find the right one for you and get out there. It can be scary to try new things and meet new people but this is about your health and your mental wellbeing. Stay connected and stay healthy.

Furthermore, there are great by-products of remaining connected to your community from combating loneliness to finding a new drive in life. No matter how you look at it, we are meant to stay connected with those around us. So make sure that this is part of your new routine. It will benefit your mind and body beyond measure.

While we are considering what community means for physical health, we should also consider the future of aging. Due to the aging population, more resources have been poured into the field and you might want a sneak peek of what to expect from future developments. Read on for an idea of what scientists have been working on. It can change the entire landscape of aging.

10

THE FUTURE OF AGING

The future of aging, like everything else these days, is changing. It's in a constant state of flux as researchers are discovering new ways to better the lives of seniors, or even lengthen lifetimes. In order to understand what to expect in the coming years, we should take a look at what the myths are surrounding the aging process. And what the science says about it. So, let's see what the future holds for us.

DISPELLING OLD MYTHS ABOUT AGING

We've already discussed how aging no longer needs to mean a loss of vitality. I have known several older individuals who stayed active and strong into their late 80s. With the right game plan, you too can experience a renewed sense of vitality in your life. Don't fall into the trap of negative thinking. There are promising studies that are revolutionizing the way we view and address aging.

Myth #1: We All Age the Same

A lot of people believe that aging is a blind process. Everyone is affected the same. In fact, old age is characterized by diversity. While some in their 60s and 70s might struggle with cognitive impairment or mobility limitations, others might have mental faculties and fitness levels comparable to one in their 30s. There is no "one-size-fits-all" model of aging so don't limit yourself.

With the new studies into how fitness and eating right factor into aging, we can therefore conclude that by following these life-style changes, your aging process will look quite different from someone who lives a more sedentary and unhealthy lifestyle.

Myth #2: Most Older Adults Are Dependent on Others for Care

There is a common misconception that most elderly adults as a whole are dependent on their family members or assisted living to care for them. This is simply not the case. In fact, around the world, only a small proportion of older adults necessitate this kind of care. It has been found that a great many older adults are living their lives independently now, shopping for themselves and taking care of themselves.

This means that there is hope that assisted living might not be around the corner for you. However, if you find yourself as someone who requires some extra care, do not carry shame for this fact. There is a wide demographic within the older population and not everyone responds to the aging process the same.

Myth #3: Population Aging Will Impose a Great Financial Burden on the Healthcare System

This myth needs to be put to bed. Not only is it not factual—it is dangerous. We needn't stress about what our aging *might* be costing the average healthcare consumer or the healthcare system as a whole. Yes, there is a slight uptick of financial burden as the population's age grows longer. However, it is not as substantial as we have been led to believe. Although old age is generally associated with the need for more healthcare, in reality, the link between age and health care utilization is weak.

For instance, in low-income settings, despite the risk of disease in those areas, older adults tend to use health services *less* than younger adults would. In high income areas, the studies also show a drop off of health care usage around 70.

While this is good news for the industry, it also points to a problem. This should also serve as a reminder to you that you are allowed to take up space. Don't feel like you are a burden.

Myth #4: Good Health is the Absence of Disease

Okay, hear me out on this one. It might sound a little bit out there. After all, we regard disease as the antithesis of good health. However, it is possible to still live an active and healthy life with a chronic illness or disease. Somewhere around 70 percent of older adults are living with some kind of illness such as heart disease or diabetes. This does not eliminate you from healthy living. You can still live a good and healthy life, despite these health struggles.

If you find yourself as one of the 70 percent, take heart in knowing that your life is far from over. There are definitely considerations you have to take into account when you are living with a chronic ailment. However, you can *still* enjoy health benefits from exercising safely and eating right. Living with diabetes might seem like a prison sentence but in actuality, thousands are living with the illness who are the picture of health, eating right, and going to their local gym regularly. Don't let a health label limit you.

Getting Rid of Those Pesky Preconceived Ideas

As you rid yourself of these myths and mistaken notions that do not serve you, you can start looking at aging through the correct lens. With these facts at your disposal, it is my hope that you can find renewed hope in the aging process and better understand how it will truly look.

You are your own best advocate. Make sure that you fully understand the *truth* behind aging and use that to your advantage. Don't limit yourself to outdated myths and half truths. Instead, see beyond the old wives' tales and understand the facts about aging. If you wish, there are great books on the subject that you can check out at your local library.

The important thing is to understand your own aging process and determining that it will look different from those of others. There is no one-size-fits-all process when it comes to aging so don't play the comparison game. This will only feed into more myths and preconceived ideas.

WHAT THE SCIENCE SAYS

Now that we have dispelled some of these old myths, it is time to move forward and see what science has to say about the aging process—more to the point, the future of aging. There have been some enlightening studies done recently that can help us understand what the future holds. As we have noted earlier in this book, eating the right foods and exercising can help you look and feel years younger. That does not need to be repeated. I think we have reached the point where you fully understand.

However, there have been other breakthroughs in the field of aging that bear a closer examination in this chapter. For instance, there has been a promising study on the diabetes drug Metformin. Though it is commonly used for the treatment of diabetes, it has been shown to work on the mechanics of aging as well. The drug can slow not just the progression of diabetes but of many age-related illnesses.

When we look at a drug like this, that has been around for some time, and see how its usage is being viewed in a new light, we can find hope. There might be other drugs on the market right now that could potentially be an age-defying miracle. The studies don't stop with Metformin, though.

There has also been an interesting finding in the field of insulin —not the drug but the commonly produced substance within your body. It was in a Florida-based research facility that scientists discovered something remarkable with major ramifications for longevity research. As stated, the study focused on insulin, a hormone that signals to cells to pull in glucose from the blood. This process keeps blood sugar in a safe range and helps maintain energy for the body.

Now, even before this study began, scientists were aware of the connection between insulin and the regulation of longevity. Unregulated signaling (electric pulses delivering messages in the body) has been shown to cause a reduced lifespan, while reduced signaling can extend the lifespan. Now, comes the interesting part.

These Floridian researchers discovered a 'decoy' insulin receptor in roundworms that is essentially a truncated version of the original receptor. The decoy is secreted into areas surrounding the tissue of the worm, effectively capturing insulin molecules before they can complete their task of signaling. What the researchers realized was that overproduction of the decoy increased the worm's lifespan.

From this research, they were able to deduce that if humans were to have decoy insulin receptors and their production was increased, they could expect a longer lifetime. This is a huge breakthrough in the possibility of lengthening a life span. However, it is still in the developmental phases and the researchers are working on a way to implement their findings in a human system.

Though this research is still relatively new and still developing, it shows that there is still so much we are learning about aging in the human body. Researchers are determined to find ways to extend one's lifespan and with this research, they are on the right track.

Furthermore, medical science is not just interested in the longevity of life but the *quality* of life, as well. That is why researchers have honed in on illnesses related to aging, such as arthritis. As of right now, over 23 million people in the United States are suffering from osteoarthritis, a condition that develops as one ages. By finding ways to prevent and treat this condition, the quality of life for millions will improve exponentially.

According to researcher Martin Lotz, MD, "Over the past two decades, we've learned a great deal about what aging is at the cellular level. What we are finding is that there are commonalities among the various tissues of the body and that ideas for preventing degeneration in one organ or tissue may be applicable to others." This is huge news for those suffering from chronic pain in the midst of their aging.

For instance, Lotz noted that in both neurodegenerative diseases and osteoarthritis, the process called autophagy—the process of disposing of old and malfunctioning cells—is thought to be disrupted in the elderly. This janitorial function declines with age, leaving these aged cells present in the body, generating toxic, inflammatory substances that damage other types of tissue. In order to study this process and how to prevent the breakdown, Lotz has focused on several key proteins.

These proteins play a key role in the maintenance and repair of cartilage. One in particular that he honed in on was that of FOXO. Lotz and his fellow researchers studied FOXO activity in cells from the shock-absorbing structures in the knees. Through these studies, they discovered that those with osteoarthritis showed abnormal FOXO activity compared to those without osteoarthritis.

From these findings, Lotz and his team of researchers are hopeful that they can design a special compound that can slow the effects of degenerative diseases like osteoarthritis. While it is still in the developmental stages, they are working alongside pharmaceutical companies to make sure that this discovery can forever change how arthritis is handled by the medical field, providing relief to the aging population.

Furthermore, there have been great strides in detecting illnesses before they actually develop. In the past, we only had a family history and a shot in the dark to determine if someone would develop certain genetic illnesses. However, in recent years, genetic testing has completely changed the game.

Current genetic testing is now affordable and accessible, allowing people to determine exactly what diseases they run the risk of developing. I'm sure you have heard of the home genetic testing kits such as 23 and Me. These kits are not only great for figuring out your family tree. They also have features that allow you to see the risk you carry for developing certain illnesses. This can be a great way to begin preventative measures before the illness has a chance to develop.

According to Ali Torkamani, Ph.D., director of Genomics and Genome Informatics at Scripps Research Translational Institute, "When you know your genetic disease risk, you become empowered to change your trajectory to live a longer and healthier life" (*The Future of Healthy Aging - Scripps Research Magazine*, 2021). With better knowledge of what you may be facing, you can start to prepare. If heart disease is something that is known to be evident in your DNA, you can attempt to live a more heart-healthy life before you even start to feel the effects.

With all of these incredible strides taking place in medicine right now, it is hard to predict what researchers will come up with next. However, I hope by reading about these breakthroughs, you are left with a bit of hope when facing the aging process. I have said it before and I will say it again—you are your own best advocate. With the right knowledge about the changing science of aging, you can better help yourself. So, stay informed. It can change everything.

WHAT THE FUTURE LOOKS LIKE

It's true that no one can fully know what the future holds. However, current studies can give us an idea of what to expect regarding aging. With DNA kits like 23 and Me so popular right now, researchers have more data than ever before to work through genetic mysteries. If you haven't already, I greatly recommend procuring one. Not only can it give you an idea of what to expect in your own future, but you can also contribute to wider studies regarding those potential disorders.

Furthermore, you can expect to live longer if you view your own aging process with more positivity. This can be difficult with agism and realizing all the changes you're going through. However, it has been found that adults who view the aging process with positivity live, on average, 7.5 more years. That's a sizable boost from just thinking about things a little differently. Change your lens and you might find that your life is lengthened by years.

As shown in the previous section, there is a lot to feel positive about. Great strides are being made in the science of aging that could change your entire life, in your lifetime. As the population grows older with longer life expectancies, much study has gone into quality of life for aging adults. This means that you could see yourself reaping the benefits of these studies even in the near future.

The fact of the matter is, what was once mysterious to researchers has begun to emerge with more clarity. Illnesses like arthritis have become a research priority as the population continues to grow older. With the studies currently being done, we could expect to find clinical answers to prevention and treatment. This is good news for the aging population.

However, we must also look at other factors that can impact quality of life. For instance, Alzheimer's is an illness that affects 3 million people any given year, and it affects the mental faculties of the individual. It is a devastating illness that can include confusion, memory loss, and inability to care for oneself. However, due to the increasing number of diagnoses, more resources have been put into discovering a way to prevent and treat it.

Currently, Alzheimer's medications work by temporarily improving symptoms of memory loss and cognitive effects. How they create this effect is by boosting chemicals in the brain responsible for carrying information from one brain cell to another. However, at the moment, these medications fall terribly short. They do nothing to slow the decline of the brain. As more cells die in the brain, Alzheimer's Disease continues to progress. The current medications do nothing to stop this cell death.

However, researchers are currently hopeful about the strides they've made in their studies. They hope that soon, drugs will be able to target the dying cells, delaying or stalling their death, halting Alzheimer's in its tracks. As understanding of how the disease works has led to change in treatment plans, looking at medications that short-circuit basic disease processes has become the new frontline approach.

The future of treating Alzheimer's will likely include multiple pharmaceuticals to combat the disease, much like you would see with cancer or HIV. Some of the treatments currently being developed seek to target clumps of the protein beta-amyloid (plaque). These plaques are characteristic signs of Alzheimer's making itself known in the brain.

There are several strategies aimed at this particular protein that seek to not just momentarily suppress symptoms but stop the disease in its tracks. One such tactic is to recruit the immune system. Several drugs, known as monoclonal antibodies, may keep the beta-amyloid proteins from clumping together into plaques, effectively stalling the progression of the disease. Others still seek to remove these plaques from the brain, setting the disease back. Currently, the studies surrounding this particular treatment are extremely promising and have entered into phase three trials.

Furthermore, there is a drug that has been around for a while, initially used to fight off cancer. This drug, known as saracatinib, is currently being tested for Alzheimer's treatment. During experiments with the drug, saracatinib turned off a protein that allowed synapses to start working again in mice. The animals subsequently experienced a reversal in memory loss. Human trials for this drug are now underway and we could see it hitting the shelves in our lifetime.

It doesn't stop there, though. Researchers have been throwing everything and the kitchen sink at the problem, intent on finding a long-term solution to the problem of Alzheimer's Disease. These dedicated researchers are also looking at the part that inflammation plays in the disease.

Since this disease causes chronic, low-level inflammation of the brain cells, researchers have honed in on this fact to search for a solution. They have begun researching inflammatory processes at work in the brain to find the best way to combat the development of the illness. The drug sargramostim—also known as Leukine—is currently in research. It is theorized at this time that the drug can stimulate the immune system to protect the brain from harmful proteins.

There are a variety of different therapies being tested and considered as these researchers move forward with their studies on Alzheimer's Disease. What they have found is hope. There is hope that a cure is around the corner. Now that they have pinpointed problem areas that can lead to the development and progression of the disease, they have a better grasp on how to halt it in its tracks.

As research develops, we will see ways in which we can live our lives as healthy and active adults. It isn't all about disease prevention, though that can be a great goal for researchers. It is about understanding the path forward. As more research comes out about the aging process, you will be able to take greater control of your health and forge ahead.

THE BOTTOM LINE

There are a great many myths about aging that can trip us up and leave us feeling discouraged about the process. However, we need to dispel those old myths and march forward with hope and the right information. The truth is, science is optimistic about the future of aging. And you should be too! Just a positive outlook can lengthen your life, so keep that in mind when you are considering your aging.

Furthermore, science is coming a long way in creating a better quality of life for the older population. As the population's lifetime continues to lengthen, we are at a place in history when aging science has become a major priority. We don't want to just lengthen life but make it worth living.

Through these studies, we have seen great progress in the treatment of illnesses like arthritis and Alzheimer's disease. There is no telling what other developments are around the corner to make life just a bit easier for those who are older. Remain hopeful, and remain active. You are, I'll say it again, your own best advocate. So, keep your own health in mind and ensure that you see your general practitioner on a regular basis.

CONCLUSION

Aging is an unavoidable part of living. In fact, you should be celebrating the fact that you have made it this far! It is a commendable thing to have lived as much life as you have lived. Take time to revel in that fact and look around at the blessings in your life. Some of them might surprise you. While aging is inevitable, loss of vitality is not. You have what it takes to forge your own path of strength and health. You have started the process in the right place, by picking up this book.

The fact of the matter is—you are starting to take your health more seriously and this is a good thing. You want to have more time and more energy to spend with the ones you love. Making this a priority gives you motivation to keep going, even when the going gets a little tough.

However, I think I have made my point abundantly clear—exercise and eating right is not just an option at this juncture. It is imperative to your health. I have regaled you with study after study that shows the innumerable benefits of proper nutrition and staying active. I don't have to go back over it but I do want to remind you that these studies are backed by legitimate science.

When you make these choices, you are making your health a priority and you will begin to see the benefits.

It can be difficult to make these changes in your life. I understand that. We are set in our ways and change can be hard. However, when it comes down to it, you need to remind yourself of the motivation behind the action. As I mentioned earlier in this book, it helps to remind yourself of *why* you're doing this. Perhaps you want more time to spend with family. Maybe you want more energy to run around with the grandkids. Whatever your reasoning, make sure you always have that in the forefront of your mind as you work towards this health goal.

Furthermore, don't feel like you need to jump into the deep end right away. In fact, it is better if you take small steps toward your goal. You are less likely to become overwhelmed this way. So start with something small like taking a walk around your neighborhood in the mornings and work your way up from there.

When deciding what to eat, make sure that you are seeking out the proper nutrients that your body needs as you age. However, remember that this needn't be a chore. You can still enjoy the food you're eating. You just have to get a little creative. If you are having a hard time with this, there are quite a few meal prep plans you can subscribe to that can help make meal planning a little easier.

Remember as you go through this change that everything is connected. Your body and mind are part of the same being. So, as you are exercising and eating right, allow yourself to do some much-needed self-care. Take care of your mind as well as your body. Remember to practice your mindfulness exercises and to stay connected with others. There are dozens of ways you can care for your mind as you care for your body. Simply make that another priority. (I swear, I'm not trying to overwhelm you.)

Finally, remember to stay connected to those around you. It is vitally important that we as a species continue to grow *together*. Combating loneliness can be a difficult process but the chapter concerning community laid out some great practices for staying in tune with the local (and distant community). Return to them when you need fresh ideas, as community is one of the most important things to have in your life.

Now it is time to put these techniques into practice. Take the knowledge that I have imparted to you throughout this book and give this your best effort. Your vitality is not something to be ignored as you age. Instead, keep an open mind about trying new things and exploring new avenues to keep your mind and body active.

It is my hope that this book gives you not only practical steps to health, but belief that it is possible. We have a good idea of what the future has in store in terms of aging. With this in mind, we can make the right choices here and now to give ourselves the best shot at a long, healthy life. I wish you the best of luck on your journey and hope that you return to these pages whenever you need some additional support. You've got this! Now, go out and live the best life you can.

I believe that you have it in you to make these changes and live the life befitting one with such grit and wisdom. So, go forward and make the right choices, for yourself and for those whom you love.

REFERENCES

Aims Healthcare. (2021, June 10). *Why We Should Care For Our Elders. Aims Healthcare.* https://aimshealthcare.ae/blog/why-we-should-care-for-our-elders/

Breeding, B. (2018, July 23). *Positive Aging: Changing Your Mindset About Growing Older.* MyLifeSite. https://mylifesite.net/blog/post/positive-aging-changing-mindset-growing-older/

Dietary supplements for older adults. (2021). National Institute on Aging. https://www.nia.nih.gov/health/dietary-supplements-older-adults

Fetters, K. (2019, April 24). *9 best types of exercise for older adults.* SilverSneakers. https://www.silversneakers.com/blog/best-exercise-older-adults/

Garza, A. (2016, January 19). *The aging population: The increasing effects on health care.* Pharmacy Times. https://www.pharmacytimes.com/view/the-aging-population-the-increasing-effects-on-health-care

National Council on Aging. (2021, February 23). The National Council on Aging. Www.ncoa.org. https://www.ncoa.org/article/healthy-eating-tips-for-seniors

Nurse Next Door. (2019, May 13). *Six important roles of the older family member |.* Nurse next Door Home Care Services. https://www.nursenextdoor.com.au/blog/six-important-roles-of-the-older-family-member/

Pajer, N. (2021, October 21). *30 of the best anti-aging foods to make sure you are incorporating into your diet.* Parade: Entertainment, Recipes, Health, Life, Holidays. https://parade.com/1170425/nicolepajer/best-anti-aging-foods/

Senior Lifestyle. (2020, February 4). *7 Best exercises for seniors (and a few to avoid!).* Senior Lifestyle. https://www.seniorlifestyle.com/resources/blog/7-best-exercises-for-seniors-and-a-few-to-avoid/

Seniorlink. (2020, May 11). *6 Benefits of Swimming for Seniors*. Www.seniorlink.-com. https://www.seniorlink.com/blog/6-benefits-of-swimming-for-seniors

Seventy is the new 50: Why our lives are different today. (2020, February 25). After Fifty Living. https://www.afterfiftyliving.com/70-is-the-new-50-why-our-lives-different-today/

Ten of the best supplements for healthy aging. (2021, September 9). Healthline. https://www.healthline.com/nutrition/10-of-the-best-supplements-for-healthy-aging

The future of healthy aging - Scripps Research Magazine. (2021, July 20). Scripps Research Magazine. https://magazine.scripps.edu/features/2021/summer/the-future-of-aging/

Thorp, T. (2018, June 29). *You're never too old to change: How to develop new patterns at any age*. Chopra. https://chopra.com/articles/youre-never-too-old-to-change-how-to-develop-new-patterns-at-any-age

ABOUT THE AUTHOR

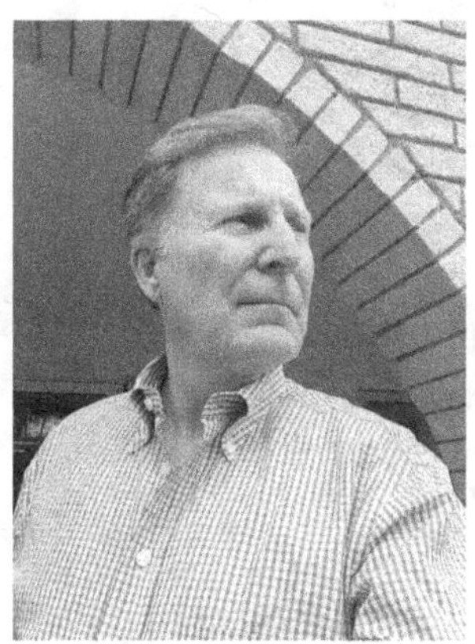

Will Anderson has been a journalist for four decades, covering major stories around the globe. He is a former television producer (The Power Boat Television Show) of lifestyle programming, interviewer, broadcaster, and podcast producer.

Will lives in Niagara on the Lake, Ontario.

www.ingramcontent.com/pod-product-compliance
Lightning Source LLC
Chambersburg PA
CBHW071040250726
48653CB00005B/1918